AVOIDING MEDICAL ERRORS

AVOIDING MEDICAL ERRORS

One Hundred Rules
to Help You Survive Mistakes
by Doctors and Hospitals

Robert M Fox
Chris Landon

ROWMAN & LITTLEFIELD
Lanham • Boulder • New York • London

Published by Rowman & Littlefield
An imprint of The Rowman & Littlefield Publishing Group, Inc.
4501 Forbes Boulevard, Suite 200, Lanham, Maryland 20706
www.rowman.com

6 Tinworth Street, London SE11 5AL

British Library Cataloguing in Publication Information Available

Library of Congress Cataloging-in-Publication Data

Names: Fox, Robert M, 1925–, author. | Landon, Chris, 1951–, author.
Title: Avoiding medical errors : one hundred rules to help you survive
    mistakes by doctors and hospitals / Robert M. Fox, Chris Landon.
Description: Lanham : Rowman & Littlefield, [2020] | Includes biblio-
    graphical references and index. | Summary: "Preventable errors by
    doctors, hospitals, and other healthcare providers are a major cause of
    death and disability in the US, comparable to cancer and heart dis-
    ease. The rules explored in Avoiding Medical Errors help patients
    avoid becoming victims and address areas that might otherwise be
    overlooked"—Provided by publisher.
Identifiers: LCCN 2019051345 (print) | LCCN 2019051346 (ebook) |
    ISBN 9781538135716 (cloth) | ISBN 9781538135723 (epub)
Subjects: LCSH: Medical errors—Prevention. | Accidents—Prevention.
Classification: LCC R729.8 .F69 2020 (print) | LCC R729.8 (ebook) |
    DDC 610.28/9—dc23
LC record available at https://lccn.loc.gov/2019051345
LC ebook record available at https://lccn.loc.gov/2019051346

∞ ™ The paper used in this publication meets the minimum requirements of American National Standard for Information Sciences Perma-
nence of Paper for Printed Library Materials, ANSI/NISO Z39.48-1992.

To all patients, wherever they may be.

CONTENTS

ACKNOWLEDGMENTS

First, and before all others, I thank my wife, Isabelle, for her understanding, patience, and assistance during the years I worked on the "rules." She was a valuable sounding board through draft after draft. My coauthor and friend Chris Landon carefully reviewed each rule; his insight and comments were much appreciated.

Many others—both professional and lay communities—provided help and encouragement. Although there are too many to name and thank, I would like to single out two of them: John T. James and Mark Scholz.

John T. James, PhD, retired chief toxicologist of the National Aeronautics and Space Administration, is the author of a detailed and carefully researched study of deaths due to errors in hospitals: "A New, Evidence-Based Estimate of Patient Harms Associated with Hospital Care." This study was published in 2013 in the *Journal of Patient Safety* and elsewhere and supplied important foundational evidence for the entire patient-safety movement in the United States. This includes the landmark July 17, 2014, Senate committee hearing headed by Senator Bernie Sanders: "More Than 1,000 Preventable Deaths a Day Is Too Many: The Need to Improve Patient Safety." Dr. James was very supportive of our interest in the patient-safety movement and rules concept. He encouraged us, and we thank him.

My thanks, also, to Mark Scholz, MD, medical director of prostate oncology specialists in Marina Del Rey, California, and executive director of the Prostate Cancer Research Institute. I am very grateful to Dr. Scholz's support and encouragement over the years.

INTRODUCTION

THE PROBLEM: TOO MANY DEATHS

Let us imagine that two 747 jumbo jets carrying more than a thousand passengers crashed because of pilot error, killing all passengers. There would be a tremendous national uproar—government investigations, a media frenzy, litigation by families of dead passengers—and the outcry would be deafening and continuing. Then the next day, let's say that two more 747s crash, again killing more than a thousand passengers. And let's suppose that this goes on—day after day—for the entire year; more than a thousand people die each day due to pilots' mistakes.

You are probably thinking that there is no way this could happen. Yet this is exactly what goes on each day in the United States—*but not to airline passengers.* More than a thousand patients in the United States now die in *hospitals* each day—more than 365,000 each year—because someone in the hospital (a doctor, nurse, technician, or someone else) makes a mistake that could be avoided. These *preventable errors*, and the terrible resulting death toll, have received:

- Almost no media attention
- Little discussion by government or private sources

- No talk show discussion by "experts"
- No screaming headlines in the daily press
- No television appearance by our president—or any other government official—to reassure the public and promise prompt action to stop these unnecessary and avoidable deaths

There are several reasons why there has been a "wall of silence" concerning these tragedies, with almost no public recognition or discussion:

- Unlike an aircraft crash, these deaths do not occur dramatically at the same time and place. They occur quietly at hundreds or thousands of different hospitals scattered all over the United States, and they occur at different times of the day and night. Many are not even reported in the local press. Knowledge of the deaths is generally unknown except for the families and hospital personnel involved. Only rarely—if a celebrity is involved—does the death even become known and attract local or national attention.
- Such deaths are rarely reported or recorded as occurring due to preventable errors. There is understandable reluctance by doctors, hospitals, or "risk management" personnel to either admit or record any evidence of wrongdoing.
- None of us, including the families and others who know of these deaths, want to believe that doctors and other health-care providers could be responsible for so many preventable deaths. Most us want to trust our doctor. We like to think of our doctor as an all-wise parent. Throughout the ages, we have relied upon those with special wisdom and powers— from ancient medicine men to the highly qualified and trained specialists of modern medicine. Our tendency is to passively trust and retain faith in our doctors. We feel unqualified to solve our own medical problems and are reluctant to criticize or think negatively about our doctors. For most of us, medical diagnosis and treatment are a mystery.

This attitude is understandable because we rely on doctors to make life-and-death decisions. We want to believe and to trust that they will wisely and safely treat us.

But on July 17, 2014, some grim, disturbing, and convincing facts came to public attention that should compel all of us to reevaluate our faith in the integrity and safety of our medical system. On that date, in Washington, DC, witnesses testified before the US Senate Subcommittee on Primary Health and Aging, chaired by Senator Bernie Sanders of Vermont. The title of the hearing was "More Than 1,000 Preventable Deaths a Day Is Too Many: The Need to Improve Patient Safety."

The witnesses at the all-day hearing were leaders in the United States medical, academic, and public health community. They included the following:

- Peter Pronovost, MD, an internationally recognized authority on hospital and medical care. Dr. Pronovost is the senior vice president for Patient Safety and Quality, and he is the director of the Armstrong Institute for Patient Safety and Quality at Johns Hopkins Hospital in Baltimore. In his 2010 book *Safe Patients, Smart Hospitals*, he states: "Hundreds of thousands of patients will die each year as a result of medical errors. Well-intentioned doctors leave instruments in patients, overdose children with medications, and operate on the wrong side of the body." Dr. Pronovost used the example of the two daily crashes of 747 jumbo jets to dramatize the problems faced by hospital patients in the United States.

- John T. James, PhD, retired chief toxicologist of the National Aeronautics and Space Administration. Dr. James is the author of a detailed and carefully researched study of death due to errors in hospitals. His study, titled "A New, Evidence-Based Estimate of Patient Harms Associated with Hospital Care," was published in 2013 in the *Journal of Patient Safety* and elsewhere. Dr. James concluded that there are approximately 440,000 preventable adverse events "that contribute to the death of patients each year from care in hospitals. This is roughly one-sixth of all deaths that occur in the United States each year." Dr. James also states that this problem (preventable adverse events) "must emerge from behind the 'Wall of Silence' and be addressed for the sake of prolonging the lives of Americans."

- Ashish Jha, MD, MPH, professor of health policy and management, Harvard School of Public Health.
- Tejal Gandhi, MD, MPH, president, National Patient Safety Foundation; associate professor of medicine, Harvard Medical School.
- Joanne Disch, PhD, RN, professor ad honorem, University of Minnesota School of Nursing. In her testimony, Dr. Disch also pointed out that there are not only one thousand preventable deaths per day, but also ten thousand serious complications per day.
- Lisa McGiffert, director, Safe Patient Project, Consumers Union, Austin, Texas.

All of us owe a huge debt to Senator Sanders and his committee, and to the courageous witnesses who testified at the Senate hearing. Senator Sanders noted that medical errors, causing over one thousand deaths per day, are the third leading cause of death in the United States, along with heart disease and cancer, each of which cause over 500,000 deaths annually.

WHAT PATIENTS CAN DO—ACT!

Thanks to the 2014 publicity and valuable information supplied by the Sanders Senate committee and its witnesses, this "wall of silence" has been breached and action can now be taken to address this problem and attempt to reduce the terrible death toll of 400,000-plus deaths per year caused by preventable errors. We cannot afford to wait for remedial action from government or private medical sources, although we do hope they will act on this wakeup call for help. All of us are either patients or prospective patients, and despite our understandable desire to trust and rely upon our doctors, it is clear that faith and trust are not enough. Our book was written to empower patients, despite their lack of medical knowledge, to take concrete and constructive steps—now—to reduce the terrible death toll caused by preventable medical errors. Our rules are simple to follow and can help to save the lives of you and your loved ones. Using nontechnical language, we explain what patients can do to protect themselves and to avoid becoming victims of preventable errors: Follow simple rules, ask questions, and use common sense. *No medical knowledge is needed!* Here are some of the topics we cover:

- How to locate—or be referred to—a competent doctor
- When to question your doctor's medical advice
- How to obtain an independent "second opinion"
- Questions to ask your doctor
- When and when not to follow your doctor's advice
- What to do if you feel that your doctor is not competent
- How to easily keep (and retrieve) medical records of tests, reports, and other documents so you can quickly provide accurate information to your doctors to protect your health
- Why courtesy and diplomacy by you is so important to protect your health
- What to do in the hospital to make sure you receive medications prescribed by your doctor for you and not for some other patient
- What to do if you are a hospital patient and have a 3:00 a.m. emergency and no one will come to help when you press your call button
- How to immediately obtain help in the hospital if you have an emergency
- How to have help available 24/7 in the hospital without paying the thousands required for around-the-clock nursing care

- What to do if an "adverse event" occurs either in your doctor's office or in the hospital
- What to do if you suffer injury, either in your doctor's office or while you are a hospital patient
- How to make sure your doctor selects a full-service hospital that can protect you 24/7 if you are bleeding, cannot breathe, have terrible pain, or face any other emergency
- How to protect yourself if your doctor has placed you in a subpar hospital
- How to handle paperwork *before* you enter a hospital and avoid signing documents that can cripple you financially
- How to make sure that your surgery will be done by your trusted surgeon and not by a student who is using you (while asleep) as a guinea pig
- How to change doctors if you are not satisfied with your doctor
- Why you should almost never accept treatment without first having a diagnosis
- How to decide if you should accept "experimental" medication or treatment
- How to decide if you should have elective surgery
- How to decide if you should have any surgery at all, regardless of your doctor's advice to do so
- What to take with you to protect your health in the hospital (a protective kit with some surprising items)
- What to tell the 911 crew if you or a loved one are being rushed to a hospital
- How to learn—in advance—what hospitals you should attempt to avoid
- What essential health information you should post in your kitchen and elsewhere in your home
- What essential health information you should carry in your wallet
- What you should do if you are told you must be discharged from the hospital, but you know you are too sick to leave

- Why you should avoid elective surgery on Thursday or Friday
- Why you should never have elective surgery on a weekend or holiday
- What warning signs you should print *on your body* before surgery
- What other warning signs you should print at home and bring to protect yourself in the hospital
- Where and where not to obtain medications and prescriptions (all pharmacies are not alike and some are outright dangerous)
- How to save big bucks by shopping and timing your deductibles (many of us have very high deductibles)
- Whether you should consider "concierge" medicine

We have made every effort to compose a book that is balanced and objective. We recognize the fact that there are millions of dedicated physicians, nurses, and others in the healthcare system who do their very best to help their patients. But the fact that there are more than 400,000 deaths each year, caused by preventable medical errors, demands that patients be alerted to protect themselves. Our rules, if followed, will help you to avoid becoming such a victim.

PREAMBLE TO THE RULES

Our rules explain how you can obtain the maximum benefit from your relationship with all doctors and hospitals and other health-care providers (HCPs), including MDs, DDSs, DPMs, PAs, NPs, chiropractors, nurses, medical techs, and others. These rules apply to your day-to-day conduct with HCPs throughout the years, regardless of whether you have insurance. The rules apply to routine as well as emergency visits, to medical offices as well as all hospitals—both inpatient and outpatient—from admission to discharge. They apply no matter where or how you happen to see a doctor. You do not need to have any medical knowledge to understand and benefit from these rules.

I

GENERAL RULES

Rules 1–32

This first chapter contains rules that apply to all doctors, health-care providers (HCPs), hospital personnel, and those who staff medical offices and laboratories. These general rules also cover other diverse subjects, ranging from record keeping to suggested patient conduct during interactions with HCPs.

RULE I. SELECT (OR CHANGE TO) A COMPETENT DOCTOR

Among all the relationships in your life, your relationship with your physician is one of the most important. During your life, your health is in your doctor's control. Consequently, the first rule deals with this relationship and how best to locate a doctor you can trust to care for you and your family. You may have already established a satisfactory relationship with a physician, and as long as that continues you need not deal with selection issues. However, in time, you may move, become dissatisfied with your present care, or need a specialist. In any case, the basic selection process is the same. This first rule is focused on selecting a primary physician, who is the first physician you see when you are ill. Generally, this would be a family practice doctor or an internist, both of whom usually handle all types of medical problems. In chapter 2 (Rule 44), we offer suggestions about selecting a surgeon, but the general approach is the same regardless of which specialist is involved. However, the specific steps to follow, in both selection and changing of doctors, depend on whether you fit in category A or B:

A. If You Have Full/Original Medicare

If you are covered by full/original Medicare, your choice is broad. All you need to do (to either select or change doctors) is to call the doctor's office and ask if the office accepts Medicare patients. Ask, "Is the doctor a Medicare provider?" Almost every doctor in the United States is. Also, remember that you do not need permission from anyone to select or change doctors. You can do this at any time. You do not need to get approval from Medicare. Nor need you say anything whatsoever to your present doctor or anyone else. In other words, there are no restrictions when you decide to select or change. Here are options for locating a promising doctor:

- Ask friends, relatives, business contacts, or any healthcare workers that you know (doctors, nurses, medical office workers, etc.), "Whom do you recommend as a good doctor?"
- Call any major or full-service hospital, or even a second-tier hospital. Hospitals almost always have their own large private medical groups with accredited physicians. This is a good source of doctors, and the medical groups operated by these hospitals usually provide doctors in both general practice and all specialties.
- Peruse the yellow pages, either online or in the telephone book. This lists all types of doctors and usually separates them by specialty.
- Search the internet. Simply go to Google, Yahoo, or Bing and type in the name of the doctor and location, for example,

"John Richards, MD, Encino, CA." Keep in mind that many physicians have their own websites. Just remember that you are reading a sales pitch, but some very good doctors have extensive and quite informative websites.

- Call your local medical association and ask for a referral.

An important reminder for those with "original" Medicare: Be sure to purchase a Medigap or *supplemental* policy to pay the 20 percent of hospital expense not covered by full/original Medicare. If you don't purchase this additional policy, you must pay the 20 percent personally, which can add up to big bucks (see chapter 7).

B. If You Have Any Other Insurance Coverage or Medical Plan (Apart from Full/Original Medicare)

Most readers will fit into this second group, which covers the many millions who are not covered by full/original Medicare but who have some other type of medical plan or insurance. Some in this group will be over 65 and eligible for full/original Medicare but do not want to pay for a Medigap policy to cover the 20 percent not covered. Such over-65 readers should enroll in Medicare Advantage, which is an excellent and less expensive program but also has some restrictions—see chapter 7. Most under-65 readers either have insurance or should plan to acquire insurance, which is simpler than it once was. Everyone, including those who are unemployed and those with severe preexisting health problems, is now legally entitled to affordable medical insurance.

All those in the non-Medicare group, however, no matter how they are insured or covered, must follow one simple requirement in selecting or changing doctors: Follow the rules of your particular plan, which are readily available. All insurance plans—Aetna, Blue Cross Blue Shield, United Healthcare, and many others—have publications, in print or online, telling members how to select or change doctors. The same applies to health maintenance organizations (HMOs) like Kaiser Permanente or Medicare Advantage programs, which supply all necessary medical and hospital services, including for those who receive care from the Veterans Administration (VA) or armed forces.

Generally, whether you are insured with an HMO or a group plan covering employees of your company (from a few people to thousands), you will be assigned to a doctor when you first enroll. You may not even be asked to select a doctor. However, all groups allow members to change doctors, although the rules vary according to plan.

Whether you select a doctor to begin with or change from one doctor to another once you are in a plan, the question remains: "How do I find a *good* doctor?" Remember your choice is limited unless you are willing to personally pay for an out-of-network doctor. You cannot follow the procedure previously discussed for those who have full/original Medicare and can select almost any doctor. The best method to use to find a doctor is to ask someone who has the same plan: "I need a doctor. Can you recommend one? Maybe your own doctor or someone else whom you might recommend?" If you have an individual policy with an insurance company and you don't know anyone else who has your particular policy, then ask your insurance carrier to supply you with a list of doctors who accept their plan. Many plans publish lists of available doctors in all specialties. Simply select one in a convenient location. Once you do that, you can check out the doctor using Google or another search engine and also run the doctor's name through your state website as suggested in Rule 2. If you are a veteran (VA patient), ask other patients you know or see at the VA facility, "Whom do you recommend? Who is good?" The same applies to members of the armed forces, which, like the VA, employ thousands of doctors all over the world (depending on where readers happen to be stationed). You may also ask nurses, secretaries, or any other employees affiliated in any way with your group or plan. They may have recommendations or information about doctors. Furthermore, don't forget that if you are "assigned" to a doctor whom you do not like, don't hesitate to change; it is not so difficult! Simply follow the rules of your plan.

Conclusion

Every rule in this book applies—equally—to all patients, whether they fall under the A or B category. Remember the basic objective: to select a doctor who will provide competent medical care.

RULE 2. USE STATE MEDICAL BOARD WEBSITES TO VERIFY THE CREDENTIALS OF YOUR DOCTOR

Once you locate a doctor, it is advisable to do some checking. Every state has a website that gives much information about doctors who are licensed to practice in your state. If practical, we advise readers to employ a doctor who is "board certified." This means that the American Medical Association has verified that he or she has received special additional medical training. This applies to all types of doctors, including general doctors—those certified by the American Board of Family Practice—as well as doctors for various specialties, such as orthopedics, neurology, OB/GYN, and others.

You can easily obtain such information about a doctor's credentials, what medical school they attended, the date of graduation, their specialty in medicine, and the current status of their medical license. Some states also give additional information, such as any disciplinary actions. Just go to your search engine and type in "MD medical licensing in New Jersey" (or whatever state you inhabit). These state websites are quite informative, and if you are at all computer savvy, they are easy to use.

RULE 3. DON'T HESITATE TO ASK QUESTIONS THAT CAN HELP YOUR DOCTOR EVALUATE YOUR MEDICAL CARE AND PROTECT YOUR HEALTH

We recognize the fact that the doctor/patient relationship can be intimidating. You may feel that requesting more information is embarrassing or implies criticism. Or you may feel you lack medical knowledge and that your best course of action is to listen quietly and meekly and just "follow orders." We disagree; we encourage you to think and ask questions. The entire rationale of this book is that despite your medical ignorance, there is much you can do to protect and improve your health.

Remember that all of us—doctors included—have good days and bad days. Your evaluation of the doctor/patient relationship is too important to be the subject of snap decisions. But after a few months or more, depending on the frequency of your visits and after you have accumulated some experience with your doctor, here are some questions you should be asking (and you may think of others):

- Do I feel comfortable calling my doctor and visiting him or her at the medical office?
- Does the doctor take my history and ask about my medications?
- Does the doctor listen, with respect, when I explain my concerns, or does he or she seem to be rushed, pressured, or preoccupied with other problems?
- Does the doctor's medical advice make sense?

RULE 4. BE COURTEOUS AND CONSIDERATE TO YOUR DOCTOR AND ALL OTHER MEDICAL OFFICE PERSONNEL

Don't irritate your doctor or anyone else in your doctor's office! You will obtain the best medical care if the doctor and other staff members like you. If you come across as demanding, hostile, or whiny, your medical care could suffer.

Just as you should expect courteous conduct by your doctor, you should also be respectful. Make it a habit to be on time; call if you are going to be late. If you must cancel your appointment, do it promptly (unless there is an emergency). Last-minute cancellation on the day of your appointment is thoughtless and irritating, and will prevent your doctor from scheduling other patients. A friendly and civil manner toward everyone at your doctor's office will go a long way to positively influence your medical care.

RULE 5. IF YOU HAVE DOUBTS ABOUT YOUR DOCTOR'S ADVICE CONCERNING DIAGNOSIS OR TREATMENT, DON'T HESITATE TO SPEAK UP AND ASK QUESTIONS

Sometimes, even with doctors you trust, you may have doubts about the advice you are given. You may feel reluctant to speak up; you may feel the doctor will be irritated by your question. But the following example explains the value of following your gut instinct and not keeping quiet.

Cassandra has a six-year-old daughter, Carolyn, who has been home from kindergarten for two days because of a cold and running nose. Carolyn had no fever and did not seem sick. But on the third day, as the cold continued, Cassandra was concerned and took Carolyn to their family physician, Dr. Armond. The medical office was very busy that morning. Dr. Armond was pleasant. He looked into Carolyn's throat, put his stethoscope on her chest, and listened. Then he said, "Carolyn's fine. Her lungs are perfectly okay. Her throat also looks okay. But let's not take any chances." He quickly scribbled a prescription on a pad and handed it to Cassandra and said, "Here's a prescription for antibiotics, just to be safe." Cassandra took the prescription, but she was worried and said to Dr. Armond, "But if her throat looks okay and her lungs are good, why should I give her antibiotics?" Dr. Armond, who had already stood up and was obviously getting ready to leave the room, stopped and said, "Well, it's only a precaution. You never know with kids."

But Cassandra persisted. She said, "Look, suppose I wait a few days and see if the cold just clears up. Is there any danger if I don't give her antibiotics right now?"

Dr. Armond thought for a moment and then replied, "Well, okay, let's do this. Keep Carolyn home for at least two or three days, and let's hold up the antibiotics. If her condition gets worse, just bring her back. But her cold may clear up on its own. Just watch her."

Only because Cassandra had the courage to ask did she cause the doctor to rethink his hasty resort to antibiotics. But, to Dr. Armond's credit, he reconsidered and demonstrated what every patient deserves: a doctor who will listen and not hesitate to make changes to avoid a possible error.

RULE 6. INSIST THAT YOUR DOCTOR TELL YOU THE DIAGNOSIS BEFORE YOU ACCEPT TREATMENT

There are dangers when a patient falls ill and then accepts treatment from the doctor before the doctor (and patient) clearly understand the underlying cause of the illness. To explain this rule, let's take the example of Jay, a thirty-eight-year-old who told his doctor, "I have a pain in my stomach that started about a week ago. It's getting worse every day."

The doctor did a quick examination. He did not order any tests. He told Jay, "I don't know what's wrong with you, but here is some medication that will help with the pain."

Jay took the medication even though the doctor had informed him that he did not have a diagnosis of the problem. Three days later, Jay was hospitalized with a ruptured appendix, which can be very serious and even deadly. Emergency surgery followed, and it was found that an infection had developed. Fortunately, Jay survived, although his recovery was more complicated and prolonged than would have been the case with a prompt appendectomy.

Jay could have avoided this medical disaster by following this simple rule: refuse treatment if there is no diagnosis. In his situation, with stomach pain becoming worse day by day, Jay should have refused the medication and promptly seen another doctor because the doctor admitted he did not know the cause of the pain (which is the same as admitting he had no diagnosis). Jay did not need to know any medicine. Jay knew all that he (or you) needed to know: his doctor was treating him without first making a diagnosis.

RULE 7. BE PERSISTENT, PARTICULARLY IF YOU'VE BEEN TOLD THERE IS NOTHING WRONG, BUT YOU KNOW SOMETHING IS WRONG

Sometimes, patients know they are ill, but their complaints are not taken seriously. But patients know their own bodies and how they feel. If this happens to you, we encourage you to persist until the doctor listens and takes action. The history of medicine is full of examples where doctors—good doctors—are simply wrong in their diagnosis or treatment (or both).

Let's take the example of thirty-nine-year-old Leticia, who noticed she had lost about ten pounds over the past few weeks from her normal weight of 120 pounds. She also noticed she was very tired despite the fact that she always got at least eight or nine hours of sleep. She went to her doctor, who examined her carefully and also conducted lab tests and told her, "Come back in a week and let's see what's what."

Leticia came back a week later. There had not been much change in her condition except she had lost another two pounds. Her doctor assured her: "There's nothing wrong with you. All the tests are normal. You're fine, so stop worrying. Go home and relax."

So what did Leticia do in this situation? Here, her doctor told her that she was fine. He did not act rushed or preoccupied. He did run tests, and in the past Leticia had always trusted him and followed his advice. Leticia gave the problem some thought, and after a few days she said to herself, "I can't help it. I simply must find out what's wrong with me. There is definitely something wrong." She made an appointment with her OB/GYN. He obtained her test results and conducted additional tests. He told

Leticia, "Look, I agree with the other doctor that the first tests don't show anything, but the tests I ordered worry me, and I'm referring you to a specialist." A week later, Leticia saw an oncologist, who ran some additional tests and found that Leticia had an early uterine cancer. Treatment began immediately.

Leticia's experience demonstrates the value of persistence. She knew there was something wrong, and she made up her mind she was going to find out regardless of well-meaning assurances from her doctor that there was nothing wrong.

RULE 8. OBTAIN AN INDEPENDENT SECOND OPINION

Because most of our readers lack medical knowledge, they must rely upon their doctors to impart sound medical advice. But ultimately you—the reader—must decide if you will follow that advice. Sometimes logic and common sense may alert you that your doctor's advice sounds wrong, or you may have a gut feeling that your doctor isn't sure of the advice he or she gave to you. Whatever the source of the reader's doubt, a second opinion may help to arrive at a logical solution.

But how to make sure the second opinion is *independent* and not influenced by conscious or unconscious factors of which you—the patient—are ignorant?

Take the example of Nancy, who has occasional bouts of severe back pain that lasts for ten days, eventually disappears, but then reoccurs six months later. She consults Dr. A, a reputable orthopedic surgeon, who advises back surgery. Nancy realizes that this is major surgery and tells the doctor that she will consider it, but also that she would feel more comfortable with a second opinion. Dr. A agrees and tells her it is a good idea to get a second opinion. The doctor says, "Here are the names of two other very qualified orthopedic specialists. I wouldn't hesitate to have either of them operate on me or my family."

So what should the patient do? We suggest two possible methods:

Method 1. Talk to a doctor who is *not* an orthopedic surgeon (specialist). This could be either a general practitioner or some other specialist who does not make his or her living doing surgery. Consider a neurologist, a physical medicine specialist, or any other doctor who does not operate. Why? Because all orthopedic surgeons (and other surgeons) are trained to think of surgical solutions. (Remember the old joke, "To a carpenter with a hammer, everything looks like a nail.") A doctor who does not earn his or her living by operating may be more open to the idea of a nonsurgical solution.

Method 2. Apart from speaking to a physician as mentioned above, if Nancy does consult another orthopedic surgeon, we would advise her to locate one on her own—not one of the two colleagues recommended by Dr. A, who are obviously acquainted with him. The colleague might find himself in an embarrassing position if he disagreed with the surgery suggestion of Dr. A. This is not a criticism of either Dr. A or his colleague; many such medical or surgical questions are highly subjective, and there can be legitimate differences of opinion. Consequently, to obtain a completely independent opinion, Nancy should select a consultant who operates at a different hospital in a different community—perhaps five or ten miles away. It is also worth the effort to attempt to select a second opinion doctor who is not acquainted with the first doctor. A practical method of doing so—prior to your actual visit—is to call and ask the second doctor, "I want to obtain an independent second opinion from a physician who does not know Dr. (give the name). Are you acquainted with (him or her)?"

We know this may sound awkward—or unusual. But we suggest that you do it to gain the important assurance that the opinion will be independent.

RULE 9. BE CAREFUL BEFORE YOU ACCEPT EXPERIMENTAL OR UNPROVEN MEDICATION OR TREATMENT

Patients should think carefully before they allow themselves to be a guinea pig for either medication or treatment that does not have a proven track record. Doctors may wish to test a new medication. Or it may be a new mechanical device enthusiastically endorsed by your doctor. Although there are exceptions to this rule—and we will discuss them—it is much safer to avoid using new medications or devices or participating in trials or investigations of such items. You, the medically unsophisticated patient, are in no position to judge the risks of participation.

An example would be a drug manufacturer who wishes to test a new medication, such as a new preparation to cure toenail fungus. The doctor is usually paid to do this, receiving a certain amount for each patient in the study. It may also require that the patient be supervised by the doctor while following a careful treatment regimen—each day for five or six months. The patient is also paid, and periodic reports are forwarded to the drug manufacturer. Although the money may be tempting, our advice would be to say no if you want to play it safe.

Another example that involves a new drug may be a *clinical trial* that is conducted by doctors who receive payments from a manufacturer in order to obtain the approval of the FDA (the federal Food and Drug Administration). These are studies that are designed to determine if the drug is safe and effective and can be eligible for sale to the general public. Again, we suggest that you exercise caution before you participate in such a study.

Studies like those described can be very helpful for the general population as well as the manufacturer. They can be completely ethical—as long as the doctor explains what the study involves and outlines the risks to the patient.

With these considerations in mind, what should you do? As a public-spirited citizen, what should you do if you are asked to join such a study? Should you say yes? Remember that the physician has a financial interest in having the patient participate and in conducting the study. He is not acting impartially as an *independent* medical adviser. It is not an easy decision.

Now, let's discuss exceptions to this "be careful before you accept" rule. There are times when you should consider accepting experimental and unproven medical treatment. One example would be a cancer patient where traditional and proven techniques have failed and the patient is going downhill or dying. In this situation, of course, experimental treatment should be considered since the alternative is death. Another exception would be "off-label" use of a medication, which, in the experience of most doctors, works very well. The Food and Drug Administration (FDA) may have approved sale of a drug for one use, but many mainstream doctors may find that it works very well for other uses not yet approved by the FDA. Of course, you—the patient—may not even know this, but if you do, we suggest that you discuss the pros and cons with your doctor, and if the advice seems logical, you should follow the doctor's advice. Common sense may dictate that you allow off-label use if it has generally been found to be safe and effective by many doctors.

We concede that our caveats concerning experimental drugs and treatment are not easy to apply. But since you—and no one else—will bear the consequences, we'll leave you with this advice: Don't make a quick decision. Use your common sense, ask questions, listen to your doctor carefully, and then ask yourself, "Should I or should I not?" If you are still not sure about participating, then follow the suggestions made in Rule 8 about second opinions.

RULE 10. CONSIDER STOPPING TREATMENT IF THERE IS NO IMPROVEMENT OVER TIME OR IF YOUR CONDITION WORSENS

George, age 50, consulted his general doctor for back pain that seemed to be traveling down one leg to his knee. The doctor ordered X-rays and said, "You must have sprained your back. Let's try physical therapy," and sent George to a physical therapist for treatment three times per week.

After the treatments began, George noticed that his back felt worse and the pains continued. He told his doctor, who replied, "Well, no pain, no gain—keep it up. It will help."

George followed his doctor's advice and continued the physical therapy, but he found that the pain continued—sometimes worse on one day than on another. But after the third week, it became even more painful, and George informed his doctor that he felt the treatment was not working. The doctor said, "Well, let's give it another week. I think that might do it, even though I know it's tough."

George continued for two more treatments and then decided he had had enough. He consulted another doctor who referred him to a neurosurgeon, who diagnosed George as having a spinal tumor that required prompt surgery.

What can we learn from this example? Answer: If, after a reasonable amount of time, the treatment does not appear to be working—or the condition becomes worse—stop and promptly obtain an independent opinion (see Rule 8).

RULE 11. DO NOT GO HOME IF YOU DO NOT FEEL OK

This rule applies to any treatment—including injections or other outpatient procedures, whether done as an outpatient at a hospital or at a doctor's office. Some of these procedures, such as a colonoscopy, require an anesthetic that puts the patient to sleep. It may be done at an ambulatory surgical center or in a full-service hospital (see Rule 41 and Appendix B). But many of these procedures have one thing in common: the patient is sent home very soon after the procedure.

We suggest that unless you feel absolutely A-OK after the procedure, there is no rush to leave the medical office, hospital, or other facility. This rule also applies even if you are comfortable walking or if there is an offer to have you leave the office in a wheelchair—and even if someone else is going to drive you home. If you do not feel quite right, simply ask to sit in the waiting room and do so for perhaps a half hour or longer until your head is clear and you feel comfortable walking or otherwise moving around.

Of course, personnel at the medical office or other facility may wish to have you leave the office. If they do, we suggest that you not argue. As long as you have someone with you, simply go outside and sit in some other nearby location—perhaps in your car in the parking area for as long as it takes you to feel okay. Then, if you do feel well, simply go home.

Take the example of Larry, who had a deep cough and went to his doctor. The doctor said, "I'm going to give you a shot that should really help with your cough. Then come back and see me next week, and we'll see how things look."

He gave Larry an injection, smiled, and said, "Okay, I'll see you in a week." The doctor left the room, and Larry stood up, ready to leave. He felt a bit wobbly as he walked out of the examining room, so he went to the waiting room and sat down. The receptionist said, brightly, "It's okay for you to go home. We'll see you in about a week." Larry started to stand. He barely made it to his feet, walked three steps toward the door, and collapsed on the floor. He was not breathing. The doctor had given Larry penicillin, to which Larry was very allergic. It is called an *anaphylactic reaction*. Fortunately for Larry, the doctor took the necessary steps to revive Larry, who suffered no permanent problems.

We learn from this rule that patients like Larry, if they don't feel well after any kind of procedure, should remain in the facility where the treatment occurred until they are comfortable. It is not necessary to know any medicine. If you do not feel okay, stay put until you do feel well!

RULE 12. TAKE ACTION—FIRMLY AND COURTEOUSLY—IF YOU ARE HABITUALLY KEPT WAITING FOR LONG PERIODS OF TIME BEFORE YOU SEE YOUR DOCTOR

Few experiences are more irritating than being forced to wait long periods of time—an hour or more—before you are actually seen by your doctor. Your time and peace of mind are just as important as your doctor's. So, what to do when—time and time again—you must wait, wait, and wait to see the doctor? You do have an option.

When you do finally see your doctor, bide your time and wait until the consultation is concluded. Then say, "Doctor, I get upset when I am required to wait an hour or more to see you. After all, my appointment time was ___, and I was here on time. Today, I had to wait almost one and a half hours [or whatever the time was]. And this happens almost every time I come. I want to remain your patient. I feel that you are a very competent doctor, and I have referred several of my friends to you. But I can't take it any longer. What can be done to handle this problem?"

In our experience, few patients make such complaints; most of us simply accept "the way it is." But there is no reason to suffer in silence. Saying nothing simply encourages such abusive conduct to continue, and it is logical to conclude that much of this behavior occurs because patients do not complain. There are many medical offices that are well organized and have short wait times—perhaps ten to twenty minutes and no more. All medical offices could be just as thoughtful—particularly if patients put sufficient pressure on doctors to act with more consideration.

RULE 13. TO SAVE TIME (AND AGGRAVATION), FOLLOW THE "CALL FIRST" AND "SCHEDULE FIRST" TIPS

Here are two simple suggestions that might also help to save you time and aggravation:

1. Call before you leave for the doctor's office and ask, "Is the doctor on time for my appointment, or should I arrive at a later time?" This may or may not help, but it is worth a try, particularly if your transport time to the doctor's office makes it feasible.

2. Try to schedule your visit so you will be the first patient in the morning or the first patient in the afternoon. This will require you to verify that you are actually the first morning or afternoon patient. But even if you are able to schedule your appointment as suggested, you can still be the victim of delay when you arrive for your "first in the afternoon" appointment. You can be told, "Sorry, the doctor is delayed because of a very sick patient at the hospital." There is not much you can do to avoid this problem except to call as we have suggested above. We also remind you that if you have a "first in the afternoon" appointment, be sure to call before the lunch hour begins so you can ask if the doctor will be on schedule for your appointment.

RULE 14. BEFORE SEEING YOUR DOCTOR, PREPARE A SHORT LIST OF QUESTIONS

Prepare no more than three or four questions or complaints that you can explain in two or three minutes to the doctor or whatever staff member interviews you. Many doctors have you first see a staff member who will summarize your concerns and record them in advance to save the doctor's time. Of course, every medical office operates differently, but the general idea is to focus your thoughts and think about your concerns in advance. Then, create a brief written list to help you tell the doctor about your concerns in no more than a few minutes. We also suggest that you ask your most important question first when you will usually have the doctor's full attention. Don't wait until the end of your visit, when the doctor may be less attentive.

Also, consider this problem: Medical costs keep rising year by year. Doctors are under economic pressure to see more patients because of simple time problems; there are only a certain number of work hours per day, and insurance companies as well as Medicare personnel are constantly attempting to hold down per-visit costs. So plan to make the most of your limited allotted time.

RULE 15. RESIST THE URGE TO TALK DURING A PROCEDURE OR EXAMINATION

When your doctor is rendering services (an examination, ECG, EEG, X-ray, CT scan, listening to your heart, or taking your pulse), resist the urge to talk; try to remain silent until the procedure or examination has concluded. Many patients wish to be friendly and almost unconsciously begin to chatter, "Nice day today," or some other small talk. But remember this rule: when doctors or others are examining you, let them concentrate on what they are doing. Do not distract their attention by talking. In other words, keep quiet until they are finished. If you don't do this, you may be contributing to possible mistakes because you are distracting the attention of the doctors from their most important task— to render you careful medical service.

Of course, after the procedure, examination, or test is over, it is perfectly appropriate to talk and ask questions.

RULE 16. IF YOU BECOME INVOLVED IN LEGAL DISPUTES, REMIND YOUR DOCTOR'S OFFICE TO PROTECT YOUR RECORDS

The main point of this rule is this: if you are involved in a legal dispute, remind your doctor and his staff to protect your records unless they have a currently dated written authorization. Routinely, you will be signing all types of authorizations from all types of entities so your medical and hospital records can be obtained.

Such authorizations may be used for Medicare, insurance carriers, and many other purposes. This rule is not intended to deal with such routine matters, but instead focuses on the very small number of patients who have ongoing legal issues and therefore need to protect their records against unauthorized disclosures. Consider the example of Joan.

Joan was injured in a serious automobile accident in which her leg was fractured because a drunk driver ran a red light. An investigator working for the insurance company—who insured the drunk driver—walked into Joan's doctor's office and said he wished to copy Joan's medical file. This investigator was simply doing his job, which was to obtain records that would help his employer—the insurance company—accomplish two objectives:

1. Find information that would enable the insurance company for the responsible driver to avoid paying out any money.
2. Obtain information about the nature and extent of the injuries of the claimant (Joan).

He presented credentials to verify that he was an insurance company representative. He told the office manager that since Joan was making an insurance claim, he was legally entitled to copy her records. The office manager asked the representative, "Do you have a currently signed authorization?" The investigator said, "No, but this is not necessary since this is an insurance matter." He was not given any information. The medical office manager was correct in refusing his request to obtain records, since he did not present the required authorization.

This rule and our example explains why signed and currently dated authorizations are important and why healthcare providers should be alerted to protect the privacy of patient records despite requests by "investigators," "adjusters," or anyone else who does not produce a currently dated authorization.

RULE 17. EDUCATE YOURSELF ON DOCTORS AND HOSPITALS

You should learn about the differences between doctors and other healthcare providers, and you should learn about the different types of hospitals and clinics. We have taken great care to explain the steps you can take to preserve your health and to survive and prosper. So it is only logical for you to take a few minutes—that's all it takes! Read Appendix A (doctors and other healthcare providers) and Appendix B (hospitals and other organizations with similar services). These explain whom you will be dealing with all during your lifetime health journey, so it will be well worth the effort. We suggest that you do a quick read of these two appendixes now; you can always go back and look again to refresh your memory. They will help you better understand and utilize the rules in our book. Also, Rule 21 explains how you may create a kitchen poster to have such information immediately available to you (or family members) in an emergency.

RULE 18. IN AN EMERGENCY THAT REQUIRES HOSPITALIZATION, BY PRIVATE CAR OR "911" VEHICLE, ASK TO BE TAKEN TO A FULL-SERVICE HOSPITAL

When you are rushed to the hospital because of serious injury or illness, via either 911 ambulance or in a private car, your best chance of obtaining proper diagnosis and treatment, and surviving, is at a full-service or "top tier" hospital. Almost all full-service hospitals have reliable 24/7 emergency rooms (ERs). But how do you obtain transport to one of these full-service hospitals and avoid the second- and third-tier hospitals? The 911 crews generally take you to the closest hospital, but little attention is focused on finding the most qualified hospital for your medical problem. However, if you know the location of either a full-service hospital or, if none is close, even a second-tier large hospital—sometimes called a *regional medical center*—you should tell the 911 crew, "Please take me to this hospital," and give the name and address. Of course, in order to do this, you must have this information readily available since emergencies do not allow research time. If you have reviewed Rules 21 and 22 (about information posted at home and in your wallet), you will have this information immediately available. What you do *not* want to do is to be taken to a "bottom" (third-tier) local hospital ER, even if it is the closest to your home. As explained in Appendix B, these local hospitals (in contrast to full-service hospitals) do not have readily available specialists (in cardiology, infectious diseases, neurosurgery, etc.). Nor do they have the facilities or personnel to properly perform complex procedures such as heart bypass surgery, valve surgery, or other complex procedures like angioplasties and stenting. These should be performed at major hospitals by experienced teams that do these procedures every single day. Another deficit of "local" hospital ERs is the inevitable delay that occurs while the patient is rerouted—usually by another ambulance—to a full-service hospital where the patient should have been taken originally.

We realize that the 911 personnel may refuse to honor your request, which would require them to spend the five or ten extra minutes required to take you to a full-service hospital. But we urge that you, along with any available family members, not give up easily; try to convince them to take you to a full-service hospital that is qualified instead of a closer third-tier hospital (see Appendix B). But if they refuse your request and take you to a lesser hospital, we suggest you relax and go with the flow. Just remember the sailor's rule: "Any port in a storm."

If 911 is not involved in transporting the patient, it is a far simpler problem: Just drive to the nearest full-service hospital, or at least one of the larger well-known hospitals. All major cities and even mid-size cities have such hospitals. The example of Tobias explains the reason for this rule.

Tobias, age 65, collapsed on the tennis court on a cool February morning. The 911 crew arrived promptly and told Tobias they would take him to the XXX Community Hospital, only five or ten minutes away. "Please don't take me to this small neighborhood hospital," Tobias said. "It has a very poor reputation and can't handle serious medical problems. UCLA is only another five or ten minutes. Please take me there." The 911 crew was reluctant. "We're supposed to take you to the closest hospital." Luckily, the tennis partner was an MD and helped persuade the 911 crew to take Tobias to UCLA. For Tobias, this was his lucky day. He had a heart attack—blockage of a coronary artery—that required immediate angioplasty and placement of a stent, a procedure done almost daily at UCLA. It was clearly far beyond the capability of the XXX Community Hospital and its personnel, who did not perform such procedures. If Tobias had been taken to the XXX Community Hospital, the inevitable delay of one or two hours, which would have been required for transport to another hospital, may have been fatal.

Reminder note: Be sure to review Rules 21 and 22, which explain how you post at home—and keep in your wallet—information about nearby hospitals and other medical notes for quick reference when an emergency occurs.

RULE 19. CONSIDER SIMPLE RESEARCH ABOUT YOUR MEDICAL PROBLEM OR MEDICATION

Whether or not you have confidence in your doctor, it is important to learn about your own medical condition and treatment. If you are willing and able to read, and/or use any computer of any kind, you can easily obtain valuable information about your health that was never available to anyone in the past, including your parents and grandparents. Here are some research and information sources.

1. The internet as accessed by your computer, laptop, smartphone, iPad, or similar device. Just type a question in the search box (Google, Yahoo, Bing, etc.). For example, let's assume you have a vision problem. Your doctor tells you that

you have a detached retina and need immediate laser surgery. You don't know anything about retinas. You access Google and type in the search box "detached retina treatment." You will immediately obtain a large amount of information. You can also go to the very comprehensive electronic encyclopedia Wikipedia, from which you will receive information in nontechnical language. You can do the same by searching information on any medication (aspirin, Advil, Celebrex) or device (laparoscope, CT scan). And the information is all 100 percent free! Other excellent sources of information include Medscape (www.medscape.com), WebMD.com, and mayoclinic.org. Avoid informal chat room information, and try to verify the information you find on more than one website.

2. Medical books written for the layman, such as the *Merck Manual* or similar books published by reputable medical organizations—the Mayo Clinic, Harvard University, Johns Hopkins, and many others. These books—often a thousand pages or more—are encyclopedic, informative, and written for laymen. You can be sure they will discuss your problem. But they can be pricey—$50 and up. Furthermore, as discussed in number 1 above, you can now obtain most of the information you need for free via the internet using any computer.

3. Medical newsletters, usually monthly, written for laymen. These are monthly publications of approximately eight to ten pages. Their cost is reasonable—$25 to $30 annually. They are usually mailed, but some are also available online. If they come from reputable organizations (universities, well-known clinics, etc.), they are very reliable. Examples would be monthly letters of the Cleveland Clinic concerning the heart, the *New England Journal of Medicine*, Tufts University's Health and Nutrition Letter, the *Harvard Heart Letter*, the *Harvard Health Letter*, the Consumer Report letter, the *Mayo Clinic Health Letter*, and many more published by major universities that are affiliated with medi-

cal teaching institutions. Simply type in any of the search bars "medical letters" or words to that effect, and your computer search engine will provide you with information about these letters: the price, subjects covered, and how to subscribe. We recommend this third option because it is inexpensive and does not require any computer know-how. Best of all, it will keep you up to date with the latest medical and health developments concerning:

- medical and surgical treatments for many different problems;
- health, nutrition, and diet tips; and
- treating—and avoiding—many different health hazards.

If medical research and reading the described information makes you anxious, simply ignore this rule and move on.

RULE 20. EVALUATE UNSUBSTANTIATED HEALTH AND MEDICAL ADVICE

We are bombarded by hundreds of health and medical tips from television, email, online ads, radio, print media, and regular mail. While there are valid sources of health information available (see Rule 19) most of the information you receive constantly from TV, radio, and print media should be either ignored or taken with a big grain of salt. These are the kinds of medical advice of which you should be very skeptical:

- Information about enhancing your sex life (usually directed at the male)
- How to lose weight
- How to avoid frequent urination
- How to treat cancer, diabetes, and many other serious diseases

- Suggested medications, ointments, and devices to eliminate pain

We hear sincere testimonials that verify the wonderful results produced. The actors employed are very convincing. Our advice: with very few exceptions, disregard these claims. They are all sales pitches, even though they may seem convincing and sincere. The advice is often unreliable and/or misleading. We suggest you obtain such advice only from your doctor or other reliable sources, such as the sources discussed in the previous rule. Consider the example of Loretta.

Loretta is overweight, and her doctor tells her that tests show she is in danger of becoming a diabetic. Loretta sees a TV ad for a new diabetic medicine "that easily controls diabetes and reduces A1c." (This is a test that helps to determine if the patient is diabetic.) She asks her doctor, Dr. Sally: "Maybe I should try this medication."

Dr. Sally replies, "Don't even think of such medication. You are only thirty-one, and all you need is simple exercise—like walking twenty or thirty minutes each day. You'll also need to cut down on bread, rolls, desserts, sugar, and sodas. You'll be fine. These 'reliable' medications can seriously damage your kidneys."

It is true that, occasionally, you might obtain valid information through television or print media. But it will be very difficult to separate the small amount of valid information from the mass of junk. We therefore suggest you remain reluctant to trust such sources unless you have very good reasons to feel otherwise.

RULE 21. IN YOUR HOME, POST INFORMATION ABOUT DOCTORS, HOSPITALS, AND MEDICATION

Emergencies occur. You may be stricken with a heart attack or stroke, or experience a serious fall or some other disaster. You may be unconscious or "out of it." Your focus should be on calling 911; this is no time for you or anyone else to frantically research or search through address books or wallets to locate vital information: What medication is needed (like nitro for your heart)? Who is your primary doctor (who should be notified)? Where is the closest major hospital where you should be taken? (See Rule 17.) To have this type of information immediately accessible to you or a family member, we suggest you simply create at least two copies of easy-to-read notices—possibly on tagboard or something else that will not easily tear. Simply use large block print on at least 8½ × 11-inch paper. For better visibility, obtain tagboard up to 18 × 24 inches from a stationery, pharmacy, or art store. But whatever the size, use a large black permanent felt-tip marker—a Sharpie or equivalent—and print the information indicated so anyone will be able to read it without glasses. Be sure to give street addresses and telephone numbers where applicable. We suggest you prepare at least two of these emergency lists, posting one in the kitchen and one in your main bedroom. Include the following information:

1. Your preferred emergency contact person (friend, spouse, adult child, or other relative). Be sure to include both land-line and cell phone numbers.
2. Your regular doctor whom you would usually contact if sick or injured
3. Specialists (other MDs who care for you, such as a cardiologist, gastroenterologist, OB/GYN, or other)
4. The closest full-service hospital (see Appendix B), as well as second-tier and smaller local hospitals
5. A 24/7 pharmacy—or two of them if they are available
6. Insurance, Medicare, or medical plan ID numbers for each family member
7. Notation of any serious allergies or food reaction problems, such as penicillin allergy or reactions to certain foods like walnuts or eggs.

Note: Items 1 through 5 are the most important for your posted notice. Readers need not feel pressured to do it all instantly, and the information for items 6 and 7 can be added at a later time.

RULE 22. KEEP MEDICAL AND PERSONAL INFORMATION IN YOUR WALLET

You may not be home when an emergency occurs, such as in the event of an accident, heart attack, or stroke. You may be unconscious or otherwise "out of it." This is why it is important to prepare a card with all of the poster information (see Rule 21) plus personal information, and keep it in your wallet, address book, or handbag. This wallet information will assist anyone who helps you, whether a doctor, nurse, family member, or Good Samaritan. Your wallet card should include the information posted at home (see Rule 21), plus additional data that is personal to you: your medication, pacemaker, stent, or any other hardware in your body—like screws or rods to hold bones together. Other family members should record similar personal information on their own individual wallet cards.

RULE 23. IF YOUR HCP OR HOSPITAL REQUIRES YOU TO SIGN AN ARBITRATION AGREEMENT, SIGN IT— AND DON'T WORRY!

It is very routine for medical personnel to ask patients, either at a doctor's office or hospital, to sign an arbitration agreement. This means that if there is a legal dispute between the patient and the hospital or doctor (usually about a medical error), the dispute will be solved by a procedure called *arbitration*, instead of going through the usual court system.

Arbitration uses the same basic procedure as the courts, but there are some significant negatives. Although arbitration may take less time as compared with court procedures, it is far more expensive since the litigants must—personally—pay the arbitrators. Also, it can be very difficult to obtain impartial arbitrators. But since you usually do not have a choice, our practical recommendation is that if you are asked to sign a hospital or doctor's arbitration agreement, do so without objection or hassle. If a dispute arises, we suggest you simply employ an experienced attorney (see Rule 104) who will know how to best navigate through the arbitration procedure.

RULE 24. CONSIDER JOINING A MEDICAL SUPPORT GROUP

It may be beneficial for you to join or form a medical support group that meets regularly and discusses medical issues either confined to your problem or general medical problems. These informal support groups are becoming increasingly popular. For example, let's say that you are a male patient with prostate cancer, or a female with breast cancer. You can search the internet for support groups in your area for those specific medical concerns. Another convenient source of information is the National Institutes of Health (www.nih.gov), which will help to locate support groups for specific diseases. Or you could speak to your healthcare provider, who may know of some support group. You can also utilize a social media site like LinkedIn or Facebook. You might also speak to other patients whom you know or find through one of your doctors. You could then suggest that you start a group—perhaps beginning with two or three patients and then increasing to some manageable number of ten or twelve—who meet once or twice a month to discuss their problems. Remember: some patients are much more sophisticated and knowledgeable than others. If you are able to put together a support group, some members will be very well informed and will help other members to gain valuable information. This will require effort on your part, but it is definitely worthwhile.

RULE 25. CREATE AND MAINTAIN YOUR OWN MEDICAL FILE

This rule may sound strange, and you may ask, "Why do this? Can't I trust my doctors to keep my records for me without my becoming involved in all this paperwork?" There are two reasons why you should physically create and update your own personal medical file, and why you cannot rely upon your doctors to maintain past and present medical information (tests, laboratory results, X-rays, MRI's, etc.).

First: To protect your health, your doctors will need your records to understand your medical history—what medications you have taken in past years, what other doctors you have seen, tests you have had and their results, all going back several years. This information should be available quickly; it should not be delayed for weeks or longer while your doctor tries to locate your records.

Second: You will see many different doctors over the years, and you may be hospitalized. If you move, your records may be in many different locations, perhaps in different cities or countries. There will be records from your general doctor, from all of the specialists you have seen, plus hospitals and laboratories. For many patients, if they have not maintained a medical file as we suggest in this rule, some of these records will be impossible to locate. Remember: doctors also may leave their practice, retire, or move to other locations. In short, unless you obtain and keep copies in your own file, many of your records will be unavailable, and your health can be endangered.

Following is a list of the records of which you should always obtain a copy and how to get them. You should read each record that you receive—for reasons we explain—and then insert the record in your medical file.

1. Obtain a copy of each prescription, whether handed to you by the doctor or sent electronically to a pharmacy or done by telephone or fax. Do whatever it takes to obtain a copy

before you give a prescription to a pharmacy or an order to a laboratory. Remember, every office now has copy machines. If it is done electronically, by fax, or otherwise, simply make sure you obtain a printout. If there is no paper copy, ask for a brief note containing the name and dosage of the medication. (You will need it for verification purposes when you receive the medication.)

2. Get a copy of each laboratory or test report for X-rays, CT scans, ultrasounds, blood tests, or any other test that the doctor orders. These reports tell what the test showed. You are legally entitled to these reports—so ask for one!

3. If the tests are digital (as are most X-rays, scans, MRIs, etc.), ask for a CD copy for your medical file. (This is in addition to the test report.) This will allow your doctor to personally review the actual X-ray or other test. Almost all laboratories now have such capability. The charge, if any, for the CD is minimal—perhaps two or three dollars.

4. If you are in a hospital—inpatient or outpatient—ask the hospital, after discharge, for a CD containing your entire record. All hospitals have this capability. Again, the cost of the CD is minimal.

5. If you are present while your doctor is dictating a report— either for your chart, for another doctor, or both—ask, "Can you please send me a copy of your report for my file?" (Be careful about this: some doctors are sensitive, and if there is any reluctance by the doctor to comply, drop it. There is no point in irritating your doctor, and you can always obtain copies of records later.)

Unless the date is clearly visible, be sure to write the day, month, and year on any medical records (including CDs) that you put in your medical file. This is essential information that may not be on your record unless you write it.

There is one more excellent reason to obtain a copy of—and read—each record: you may discover information that could protect you and sometimes even save your life. The following example of Tom explains why it is so necessary to obtain and read every document that you receive and place in your medical file.

Tom, age 40, had an odd-looking growth on his right arm. At first, he thought it was an infected pimple, but when it did not heal after two months, he showed it to his dermatologist, who removed it and said it was "probably nothing," but that it would be sent to a pathologist "to take a look." Tom asked that a copy of the pathology report be faxed to him when it came in; he gave his fax number to the office staff.

About a week after his visit, Tom went on a ten-day vacation. He had not yet heard from the dermatologist and assumed there was no problem. When Tom returned from his vacation, he found a copy of the pathology report in his fax machine. Tom did not understand the page of medical jargon, but when he saw the words "carcinoma" and "malignant melanoma" he was concerned. He immediately called his dermatologist, who told Tom, "Hold on a minute; let me see this report."

When he returned to the phone, he told Tom: "Somehow this was put into your file. I didn't see it. It's a good thing you called." He made an immediate appointment for Tom to see a surgeon and treat the problem. This example underscores the importance of asking for and reading a copy of all documents—here a copy of the pathology report. Without knowing any medicine, Tom was alerted and called his doctor when he saw the words "malignant" and "carcinoma." It probably saved his life.

Settle on one simple method to maintain your medical file (one for each year). You can use an ordinary manila file. A better solution would be a two- or three-inch expandable file that is closed on both sides so that the contents will not fall out. You could also use a standard three-ring notebook. Simply obtain a standard three-hole punch, use it for all documents, and put each in your notebook. Smaller prescriptions, notes, and any other documents can be taped to blank pages that you can also punch. As long as you put a date on each item, you will have no trouble keeping your file well organized for easy retrieval.

If there is no convenient way for you to make a copy of a document, a digital photograph—made using your cell phone—is a good practical answer. But if you do so, it is advisable to promptly make a paper copy and place it in your medical file.

Computer-savvy readers may ask, "Why do I need an old-fashioned physical file?" Our answer: It is not practical to simply record digitally all the information needed for your medical file. This is true even if you know how to use the "cloud" or some other modern gizmo. Remember that in the file for each year you have many different individual CDs or other documents, such as paper records, small slips given to you by the doctor, instructions, X-rays (also in digital form), MRIs, and others. Then, you may be handed a prescription by a doctor or receive a fax or an email or a report about some test in paper form. In other words, many of these items are not digitalized and would have to be scanned and put into digital format before you could include them on your computer, your "cloud," or elsewhere. Furthermore, many documents may be created when you are out of town, where scanning and digitalization is simply not practical.

It is far more reliable if you simply use a separate physical file for each calendar year and insert your CDs, paper documents, notes, hospital memorandums, and other items.

RULE 26. IF YOU DISCOVER AN ERROR IN ANY RECORD, ASK FOR A CORRECTIVE NOTE

You may discover an error in your medical records. For example, your name may be misspelled with a wrong first or last name, or there may be an erroneous note in your records that you had a certain disease (your father may have had a disease and your doctor may have confused you with your father—in other words, a simple misunderstanding).

So, what do you do when you discover such an error? Some doctors or hospital personnel bristle at the suggestion that they should change or alter their records. Simply make it clear that you are not asking them to make any change or alteration whatever, but that you merely wish that a *corrective note* be added with the date of the corrective note. The following example explains this rule.

Joe was in an automobile accident and explained to the doctor that the other driver ran a red light and crashed into him. Joe obtained a copy of his doctor's records before he gave permission to the insurance company to copy the record. When he looked carefully, he was disturbed to note that the record indicated that he told the doctor that he—Joe—had run a red light. Obviously, this was a misunderstanding in the taking of Joe's history. Consequently, Joe asked that the doctor make a corrective note stating, "Patient told me that the other driver ran a red light, and I make this note to correct that part of my record—Jan. 14, 2015."

We want our readers to be aware that when claims are made involving insurance companies, they make it a point to copy every single medical record they can locate. And the information illustrated in the example is exactly the kind of information they are searching for. Had Joe not asked that his doctor make the corrective note, Joe's rights could have been seriously compromised because his claim might have been denied "because you ran a red light and you admitted that to your doctor."

Of course, readers should understand we are not discussing minor errors, such as a misspelling or common typo that would obviously cause no trouble. So if it is something obviously unimportant, there is no point in irritating the doctor by demanding a correction. In other words, use your common sense and leave well enough alone unless you think the error may create some problem.

RULE 27. OBTAIN YOUR ORIGINAL RECORDS BEFORE THEIR "DESTRUCT DATE"

Medical and hospital records are not kept forever. There may be occasions when records are put on a computer and kept for years on end, but don't count on it. Most records are destroyed, erased, or otherwise eliminated after a matter of years—perhaps seven years or less. So you should take steps to obtain either the originals or a complete copy before they are destroyed. As far as your doctors are concerned—and there may be several of them—we suggest you do it both orally and in writing. Remember to be courteous and diplomatic and state (by email or an ordinary written letter): "I would like to have my original records returned before they are destroyed. What do you need from me in order to accomplish this? I will be glad to pick them up. Or you can mail them to me, or we can make some other arrangement."

The idea is to arrange something practical. But an oral request is not enough. We suggest you also send a courteous letter—as stated above—to each doctor and hospital. Be sure to provide your full name, your date of birth, and the period of time you think your records cover. If it is a hospital, try to give your hospital number if you can locate it. In addition, give the date or approximate dates you were a patient. It is advisable to remind the doctor or hospital periodically—at least by a phone call—that you have made this request and expect to have your records delivered to you or made available for pickup before they are destroyed.

It is true that what happened a few years earlier may not seem to be medically relevant when you make the request, but at some later date it could be extremely important. (An example might be the need to determine the records of several previous surgeries in order to determine when a surgical instrument was left in your abdomen.) We suggest you ask each doctor and hospital their approximate record destruct date. Then, place these items on your calendar so you can remind the doctors and hospitals at least a month before the destruct date. This will avoid the possibility of being told, "Oh, we're so sorry, we destroyed your records in error, and we forgot about your request."

RULE 28. ASK FOR WRITTEN INSTRUCTIONS FOR ANY MEDICATION, DIET CHANGE, OR EXERCISE

Many of us may be told by our doctors to take such and such a medication at certain times, daily, or before or after meals. Or other directions can be given—perhaps about foods to eat or avoid, or exercises to do. However, memory is frail, and assuming that you wish to follow your doctor's orders, we suggest you make a simple request to your doctor or the medical assistant: "Please write me a note about what I am supposed to do. That way I'll remember and there won't be any misunderstandings." If you have a recording device, ask your doctor, or a staff member, to record instructions for you. (Most smartphones will record and play back.)

RULE 29. KEEP EACH OF YOUR DOCTORS INFORMED OF YOUR MEDICATIONS AND SUPPLEMENTS

Increasingly, many of us see multiple doctors. Our general doctor (often an internist or family practitioner), perhaps a cardiologist, an OB/GYN, or a urologist. The list can go on and on.

Each of these doctors may prescribe different medications or supplements. Often, one doctor may not realize how many different doctors you are seeing during the period of a year. So, we suggest that you help each doctor to do his or her job by making sure each time you see your doctors that you keep them informed about all medications and supplements you are using. These can include medications for blood pressure, heart problems, frequent urination, cholesterol, or any other problem. And don't forget to include pain pills, such as Celebrex, aspirin, or NSAIDs. Also include all food supplements, such as glucosamine, selenium, St. John's Wort, and vitamins, to name a few. Some of these may interact with others and cause significant difficulties. Therefore, your doctors will be better able to do their jobs and protect you if they know that you are using these medications or food supplements. As we explain at Rule 32, it is a mistake to assume that doctors communicate with one another and keep one another informed. That's why it is your obligation to do so.

RULE 30. BE AS ACCURATE AS POSSIBLE WHEN PROVIDING THE DOCTOR OR HOSPITAL WITH ESSENTIAL INFORMATION

There is an old medical axiom: "Eighty percent to ninety percent of all diagnoses can be made from history alone." Consequently, when you go to the doctor or hospital and explain your problem or have a physical exam and explain your history, try to be accurate. Sometimes you will be asked to write out your medical history and complaints. Sometimes you will be asked to check various blocks or squares to tell what problems you have had. But when you fill out questionnaires, or when you describe the medical problems and your history, try to strike the proper balance between detail and brevity, but also include all essential information. Josie's example explains this rule well.

Thirty-year-old Josie had had severe diarrhea for several days. She made an appointment to see her internist and filled out the usual questionnaire about her complaints, medications, and other items. But she forgot to note that she had just returned from Mexico three days prior to her visit. It never occurred to her that this might be important.

Fortunately, when Josie talked about her diarrhea, the doctor asked her, "Has anything unusual happened in the last few weeks? Have you eaten or had anything to drink out of the ordinary?"

At that point, Josie said she just remembered she had been to Mexico and she had been "careful," but said, "I did have some ice in a Margarita." Hearing this, the doctor told Josie it was probable that she had the "turistas" and to wait a week and see if it cleared up.

That single item of history about Mexico was all the doctor needed to confirm the diagnosis and avoid expensive, unnecessary, and time-consuming tests.

RULE 31. IF THERE IS A LANGUAGE BARRIER, BRING YOUR OWN TRANSLATOR OR INTERPRETER

When you are ill or injured in this country or elsewhere, it is important to accurately communicate with your doctor. This rule applies whether you are a patient in a doctor's office or in a hospital. If you know there may be a language barrier, bring (or obtain) an interpreter; it can be a friend, relative, or anyone else. Don't worry about credentials. Usually, you don't need a licensed professional. The only requirement is someone who can understand your language and explain your problem to the doctor or hospital personnel. If a hospital insists on a licensed interpreter, they can usually obtain one—particularly a *full-service* hospital (see Appendix B). Remember that the hospital (not you) must pay for the interpreter. This is required by federal law.

RULE 32. COMMUNICATE YOUR CONCERNS TO ALL YOUR HEALTHCARE PROVIDERS; DO NOT ASSUME THEY WILL COMMUNICATE WITH ONE ANOTHER

Whether you are involved in an emergency situation (heart, blood pressure, bleeding, or other problem) or a routine medical office visit, do not assume that the doctors, nurses, and other intake personnel will communicate with one another about your medical symptoms and concerns. As we explain in the example that follows, you should make it a habit to carefully repeat your concerns, complaints, and symptoms to each HCP.

At 7 a.m., Jill awoke and found that she could not move her right arm and leg; both felt numb. She thought, "My God, I bet I have had a stroke." She called 911, and they came within twenty minutes. When they arrived, Jill told them what had happened but explained, "Now I feel better than I did when I called. At first, I couldn't move my arm and leg at all. But now I can move them, but they are weak."

The two paramedics did not seem concerned and said, "Maybe you were sleeping on your arm and leg and this made them numb." Jill replied, "No, I have never had anything like this before. I think it's a stroke."

They smiled, put her in the ambulance, and took her to the hospital, where she was admitted as a patient. She was wheeled into an ER cubicle to be seen by a doctor. She assumed the paramedics had explained to the hospital personnel her concern about a possible stroke. In addition, she assumed they had given written information about her to the admitting personnel. When the hospital attendant wheeled her into the cubicle and asked how she felt, Jill said, "Well, I'm better now." (But Jill gave no other information.)

The hospital was very busy, and it was over two hours before a doctor appeared. He smiled and asked her, "Why are you here? You look okay; anything wrong?"

She replied, "I think I had a stroke because I couldn't move my arm or leg when I woke up this morning. They are better now, but I still feel very weak."

The doctor suddenly became serious and read the notes contained in Jill's chart as well as the paramedics' notes. As he began his examination of Jill, he asked, "Did you tell the paramedics who brought you here about your arm and leg problem that you noticed when you woke up?"

Jill replied, "Yes, and I also told them I was worried that I was having a stroke, but they said that maybe I had slept on the arm and leg and caused the numbness."

The doctor replied, "Unfortunately, there's no mention in their notes about any of that, or any note that any particular complaint was made by our hospital attendant when you were admitted. This is unfortunate because we have a very specific procedure that must be followed for possible stroke victims, and action must be taken quickly. I'm having you moved to our stroke treatment area."

Jill was upset, but explained, "I assumed the paramedics would let the hospital know why I called 911—but I guess they didn't."

Jill was immediately moved to the stroke center, where it was determined that she had, in fact, suffered a stroke. But the delay in diagnosis and treatment (caused by the communication failure illustrated) caused Jill to be permanently disabled, although there was some improvement after months of treatment.

This tragedy would probably have been avoided if Jill had not assumed the paramedics would communicate her concerns to the hospital personnel. Also, had she told the hospital attendant who wheeled her into the cubicle, "I think I've had a stroke—I couldn't move my arm or leg when I woke up this morning," prompt diagnosis and successful treatment would have been probable, despite the failure by the paramedics to record and communicate about Jill's problem to hospital personnel.

2

RULES WHEN ELECTIVE OR NON-EMERGENCY SURGERY AND HOSPITALIZATION ARE FIRST CONSIDERED

Rules 33–50

All surgeries and other treatments that occur in hospitals have serious risks, especially if you are asleep or unconscious under a general anesthetic. These risks exist at our best hospitals and even with the most competent and experienced surgeons. Things can simply "go wrong" with no one being at fault. Or sometimes doctors and hospital personnel can be careless. For example, instruments or sponges may be forgotten and left inside the patient's body cavity. Patients may be administered the wrong medication or the wrong dose of the correct medication. Or surgery can be performed on the wrong parts of your body while you are under an anesthetic with no ability to warn or object (see Rules 52 and 66 about warnings by printed body signs).

These are just a few of the *preventable errors* discussed in our introduction. These facts lead us to an obvious conclusion: think carefully before you decide to have elective surgery. If you decide not to do so, you avoid the risks described (see Rule 33).

But let us not lose perspective. Each year millions of patients enter hospitals for surgery or for treatment without surgery. Most of the time there is no problem. Most patients have successful surgery or other treatment, recover, and go home.

About Emergency Surgeries

As just mentioned, the rules in this section do not apply to emergency surgeries. If you have such surgery, there is little or nothing you can do to protect yourself, with one exception. If you retain consciousness or are able to talk, simply do your best to cooperate, to be pleasant and friendly, no matter how bad you feel. When you are in an emergency situation facing hospitalization and surgery, the last thing you want to do is to be antagonistic to anyone (see Rules 4 and 63). Remember, your life is in the hands of others and you must rely upon them, so you want them in the best possible frame of mind as far as you are concerned.

We will now explore Rules 33–50 concerning both elective surgery and other surgery that is mandatory (non-elective), but which is not done as an emergency and where you have time to think, plan, and take steps to assure the best possible outcome.

RULE 33. ASK QUESTIONS AND THINK CAREFULLY BEFORE YOU AGREE TO HAVE SURGERY

Since surgery will expose you to significant risks and dangers to health and life, think carefully about this decision. Ask yourself these questions: First, why have surgery at all? Do I really need it? Is it "mandatory"—something necessary to my health and life? Is it medically necessary? Or is it elective (which is the same as optional)? If I refuse the surgery, will there be any danger to my health or life? And if elective, why have it at all in view of the real risks I will face? There may often be a real controversy. Doctor A may tell you that surgery is medically necessary and is required to maintain a good quality of life, but Doctor B may say the opposite, that the surgery is not needed (not "medically necessary").

To help you decide whether you should have the surgery, we will look at four examples. After you read and consider them and the questions that follow, you will be in a better position to decide on the surgery under consideration.

Example 1: Doctor A tells you that back surgery is needed or "you will be crippled." However, following our advice, you obtain an independent opinion (see Rule 8) from Dr. B, who tells you, "You don't need back surgery at all—at least not now and not for the foreseeable future." Dr. B prescribes treatment, including physical therapy. After a series of treatment, your back pain disappears and you are cured.

This example tells us how dangerous it can be to trust any individual doctor when you are required to make an important medical decision. The answer is clear: Before making an important medical decision, such as one involving surgery, consider obtaining a second and independent opinion (Rule 8) to help you decide. In our example, the final decision not to have surgery was correct.

Example 2: As a middle-aged woman, you find a lump the size of a pea in your right breast. You are concerned and see your doctor, who refers you to a surgeon. The surgeon cuts out the lump ("biopsy") and orders a microscopic examination by a pathologist, who looks at the lump under a microscope and tells you that the lump is cancer. Your doctor—both your surgeon and regular doctor—tell you that surgery is needed promptly in the next two weeks.

This example illustrates a very easy call. This surgery is definitely mandatory, and it must be performed. But you have a very limited amount of time to do some thinking and planning. Although you might consider a second opinion—if it can be accomplished quickly—common sense dictates your decision should be "yes" to this surgery suggestion.

Example 3: You are in your twenties and have a very long, large, and ugly nose. You may decide that "whatever the risk, it is worth it" because this nose has caused you great social distress.

Another example would be a female who has very large breasts that are causing her back pain, affecting her posture, and causing her to have a poor self-image.

Both of these examples involve clearly elective surgery, and each is probably worth the risk. But, again, a second opinion could be helpful and informative so that the patient can be fully informed about the risks as well as the advantages.

Example 4: A friend says to you, "Hey, why don't you get a facelift like I did? Get rid of those sixty-year-old wrinkles! I did it and I really recommend my plastic surgeon, Dr. Z, who is terrific." You know there will be risks if you, as a sixty-year-old, have this surgery. Yes, you have some wrinkles, but you say to yourself, "I could live with them," and you're not so sure it's worth the risk. What to do?

This is another example where a second opinion might be very valuable, particularly where such surgery is clearly elective, its dangers are probably not known or appreciated, and there would be no positive impact upon the patient's general health.

For *All* Surgeries: Ask Questions

To help you decide yes or no to surgery, we suggest that you ask each doctor the following questions. They apply to all surgeries, whether they are clearly elective or mandatory, or whether a question exists as to which classification applies. It is too difficult for any lay patient to make these distinctions and decide. Here are the questions:

1. Is there an alternative that I might attempt so I can avoid the surgery and achieve the same result?
2. What will happen if I don't have the surgery?
3. What are the risks I face if I have the surgery? And please tell me if the risk is one out of a hundred (.01), one out of a thousand (.001), or some other figure.
4. In your opinion, is the surgery worth the risk?

5. What will I gain by having the surgery?
6. How will my future be improved over the next five or ten years if I have the surgery?
7. What could go wrong, either during or after the surgery, that might cause me trouble in the future?

We realize that some of these questions overlap and seem related to others, but we suggest you ask each of them. You may learn something by asking the same question in different ways. Remember that this rule does not apply to emergency surgeries, but only to surgeries where you have time and the opportunity to think and seek a second opinion before making your decision.

To sum up, think carefully before you agree to surgery and consider this: Is it clearly medically necessary (mandatory)? If not, is it desirable for other reasons?

If you decide to have surgery, the rules that follow will help you to achieve the best possible result.

RULE 34. IF YOU DECIDE TO HAVE SURGERY, TAKE STEPS TO ASSURE THE BEST POSSIBLE RESULT

Once you have decided to have surgery, whether medically necessary or elective, you might say to yourself, "Well, I'm going to have surgery, so all I need to do is find a good surgeon, go to the hospital, and let him or her take over." Although locating a competent surgeon is obviously important, there are other essential factors and questions that you—the patient—must consider:

1. Where should I have my surgery? In my home city? Or in a city five hundred miles away where, my doctor tells me, there is a "great" surgeon with the "most experience" in performing my kind of surgery?
2. How do I look for a surgeon? Can I rely—100 percent—on my regular doctor?

3. Should I contact my local medical center, which is affiliated with a well-known teaching hospital and medical school with access to hundreds of doctors in all specialties?
4. When I locate a surgeon who seems promising, is there a simple way to find out information about him or her?
5. Do I need to do anything to prepare for our first meeting?
6. Should I ask if he or she will personally perform the surgery, or whether the instruments will actually be handled by student doctors under "supervision"?
7. Will my surgery be performed in a full-service hospital (that will allow you to have a 24/7 advocate in your room), or in a smaller neighborhood hospital where this is not permitted?

You will want to be satisfied and comfortable with the answers—to these and other questions—by your surgeon, whom you will be trusting to protect you while you are unconscious, helpless, and totally under his or her control. These questions are answered by the rules and explanations that follow.

Rules to Consider before Selecting Your Surgeon

The rules that follow (Rules 35–45) should be considered before you decide who will perform your surgery. These rules will help to answer the seven questions just mentioned.

RULE 35. AVOID TRAVELING FAR AWAY FOR A SURGERY FROM THE "BEST" EXPERT

It is definitely not wise to leave your home city—perhaps someplace like San Francisco—and travel to a distant city, perhaps Chicago or Boston. Sometimes, when surgery is to be performed, you may be told that your particular surgery would best be done by a certain renowned expert in a distant city. This advice may be given by a physician or perhaps a well-intentioned friend. But there are some very good reasons why you should stay put and have surgery done in your own home community. Assuming that you live in or near a large or medium-size city, you should be able to locate a competent surgeon, and that is where you should have your surgery—not a location hundreds or thousands of miles away.

Of course, there can be good reason to travel long distances for treatment. For example, you might live in a very remote rural area, hundreds of miles away from a surgeon experienced in taking care of your particular medical problem. Or you may live in a small town or city where your choice of surgical specialists is also limited.

In such instances, it does make sense to travel whatever distance is required. But in the United States today, such problems would be rare, because most readers probably live in or near cities that would have surgeons with the required expertise. Assuming you fit into this category, here are the reasons not to travel:

1. If there are postoperative complications, such as an infection that develops after your return home, local specialists will be very reluctant to become involved. When they are asked to treat the problem, they will very often suggest that the patient "go back to the surgeon who performed the operation. He is the best physician to treat you."

2. It will be much more difficult to arrange a 24/7 advocate to remain with you in your room (Rule 42) if you are in a distant city. Undoubtedly, you will have more acquaintances—family and friends—in your home city than you will if you travel to a city hundreds or thousands of miles away.

3. There may be a delay in discharge from the hospital if unexpected complications occur. You may need to remain in the distant city for an extra week or two, or you may need temporary care at a skilled nursing facility (SNF). This can cause family problems to multiply due to longer periods away from home, which can make it more difficult to arrange childcare or care of the home.

4. If your immediate postoperative medical condition in a distant city requires that additional specialists be called in by your surgeon, they will be unfamiliar to you. In your home city, you probably already would have a cardiologist and a urologist, and perhaps other specialists that you know. But in a distant city, you will be required to establish new relationships. Then, when you leave the distant city and return to your home city, your local specialists, if they must become involved, will have to be brought up to speed about what happened when you were away from home. For example, you may have a cardiologist or a neurologist or orthopedist in your home city, but they would be required to obtain information as to what happened when you were in the distant city for your surgery. It is far better, in order to retain continuity of care, to remain in your home city. This would avoid the problem.

To illustrate this rule, let's take the example of Alice.

Alice, thirty-eight years old, had a husband and two teenage children. She required a hysterectomy. Her friend Denise persuaded her to travel from her home in San Francisco to a "wonderful surgeon" in Chicago. Denise explained that this surgeon—Dr. Zack—"is the best there is; he did my surgery and you won't be sorry if you employ him to do yours."

Alice was convinced and traveled to Chicago. Dr. Zack was an excellent surgeon. The surgery went well, and after a few days Alice was back home in San Francisco. But the day after she returned home, she felt severe pain in her pelvic area. Her San Francisco doctor told her that he thought she had a severe infection and told her, "It would be wise for you to consult the doctor who performed the surgery. He is the doctor who should be managing your problem now."

We have outlined the problems created by Alice's decision to travel for her surgery: Dr. Zack is in Chicago, and she is back home in San Francisco. By choosing a doctor so far from her home, Alice has created unnecessary problems. Of course, she can take a plane back to Chicago, but she will then face the problems that have been discussed. Alice could have located a competent surgeon in San Francisco to perform her hysterectomy. Or Alice could have said to herself, "I wonder if I should follow my friend's suggestion to travel so far for my surgery? After all, she's not a doctor. I think I'll ask my local doctor her opinion about traveling so far from home, although I'm sure my friend's doctor is very competent."

This course of action is similar to what we advise in Rule 8, which covers second opinions. But it is much different: The friend who advised travel was not a doctor. She was simply a layperson who advised her friend.

RULE 36. VERIFY WITH YOUR SURGEON THAT HE OR SHE WILL *PERSONALLY* PERFORM THE SURGERY

It is well known that in most of the teaching hospitals in the United States, your surgeon does not personally perform your surgery despite the fact that you—the patient—have selected and employed that surgeon. He or she will—very often—supervise a resident or a fellow or intern who actually handles the instruments and performs the surgery. In other words, you—the patient—are used as a teaching vehicle. This is something you do not want to happen. You should not be a guinea pig. You can avoid this problem by having an agreement with your surgeon—when surgery is first arranged—that he or she will personally do the surgery. This should settle the issue. But the surgeon may tell you that he or she cannot or will not make this agreement, and intends to supervise others who will perform the surgery. (This may be the procedure uniformly followed at this teaching hospital.) Then you have a decision to make. Are you willing to have your surgery done by a student under "supervision"? Remember: as indicated at Rule 44, we suggest that you try to select a competent surgeon who has performed at least one hundred of your type of surgery. But if you consent to having surgery by a student, even under supervision by your surgeon, it can be very risky! You must decide if you are willing to undergo a surgery that may be the first ever performed by that student.

But let's assume that you obtain a verbal assurance from your surgeon that he or she will personally perform the surgery. While such assurance should be comforting, we suggest that certain other protective steps be taken to verify that your surgery will not be done by a student. First, carefully read the consent form that you will be asked to sign when you enter the hospital. This form usually provides that you consent to surgery by "—— [name of surgeon]—— MD." The form may have other wording (these forms vary). Such other wording usually will allow some surgeon, whom you do not know, to perform your surgery. This is precisely what you do not want to happen. Therefore, the form must be corrected to confirm your oral agreement with your surgeon that he or she (and no one else) will actually perform your operation. This correction should be done by you or your advocate quietly, without fuss, comment, or discussion with any hospital personnel. Simply cross out conflicting language and clarify that you agree to surgery performed by [insert the full name of your surgeon]. Then place your initials where you have made the correction.

To help readers make such a correction/modification in the form described, we have included in Appendix C a typical hospital consent-to-surgery form. Note that we have drawn a line through the objectionable language that would permit your surgeon to allow residents, fellows, students, assistants, or anyone else to perform your surgery. Patients should also draw lines through other similar language (these forms vary, depending upon the hospital).

After this modification has been done, at some point it is also advisable for you to reassure your surgeon that you have no objection to the use of students or others to assist during the surgery, to watch, and to learn.

RULE 37. SCHEDULE YOUR SURGERY AT A TIME WHEN THE SURGEON WILL BE AVAILABLE SEVEN DAYS POSTOPERATIVELY

Let's assume you have carefully selected an excellent surgeon and the surgery goes well. But a serious infection and unexplained bleeding develop two days after your discharge. If this happens, you will want your surgeon, who performed the surgery, to handle the problem and to treat you. It is a very simple matter. When you first employ your surgeon, ask, "Can you schedule the surgery at a time when you know you will probably be available for seven days after the surgery (post-op)?" And add, "I just would feel more comfortable if you were around if anything goes wrong." If your surgeon agrees, this should be sufficient reassurance. But you may be told, "I can't make a commitment like that; my schedule won't permit it." Then, you have a decision to make. Should you take your chances with this surgeon or find another surgeon who will make such a commitment?

It is true that generally you do not have problems after surgery if it is properly performed, and of course, the very reason you chose the surgeon is because you had confidence in this person. But we are attempting to protect you against the unusual. It is well known that after surgery, infections can develop, even though the surgery is done at a full-service hospital and by a very competent surgeon. Such a complication can occur regardless of the competence of your surgeon. In view of such risk, and the considerable effort required to locate and employ a competent surgeon, why should you take a chance on any complication being handled by a complete stranger whose qualifications you will not have the opportunity to check?

RULE 38. SCHEDULE YOUR ELECTIVE SURGERY FOR A MONDAY, TUESDAY, OR WEDNESDAY MORNING (IF YOU HAVE A CHOICE)

Things can go wrong in the best hospitals and with the most competent surgeons. If you have surgery on Thursday or Friday, and if an infection develops, it can often take a day or two to become apparent. For example, let's say you have a hysterectomy on Thursday. On Friday evening, after your surgeon has left the hospital, you are suffering intense pain, and bleeding has also developed. Your temperature begins to rise, and you develop an infection that is in *full bloom* on Saturday and Sunday. Very often your own surgeon will not be on call (available) on Saturday and Sunday. The substitute doctor who sees you will not be familiar with your medical condition even though he or she will be able to read your chart. When an unexpected problem like an infection occurs, the substitute (on-call) doctor may be reluctant to take prompt action, particularly if the patient is seen on Sunday, since your surgeon will be available on Monday morning. But let's assume you are lucky enough to have a substitute doctor who realizes prompt action is required, and that an infectious disease specialist is needed. It will be much more difficult to promptly obtain such a specialist on a Saturday or Sunday.

All of these problems are easily avoided if you follow this "Monday-Tuesday-Wednesday" rule. Your own doctor and experienced specialists will be readily available. Even if your surgery is on Wednesday, there will still be two days, with a full medical staff available, to take all necessary action.

We also suggest morning surgeries—if you have the choice—because the surgical team is more alert and rested as compared with afternoon surgery, particularly if the morning surgeries were difficult and demanding.

We recognize that your surgeon may not agree to schedule your surgery as requested; he or she may explain, "I do my surgeries on Thursdays and Fridays." To resolve this type of problem, we refer you to Rules 44 and 45, which will guide you in the decision that will be required: Should you remain with your surgeon and violate Rule 44—or find another surgeon? If you do decide to find another surgeon, remember that it may take considerable time—weeks or longer. But remember: this is elective surgery, and you should feel comfortable in taking all the time needed—weeks or even longer—to find another doctor that will not require you to violate this rule.

RULE 39. AVOID ELECTIVE SURGERY WHEN RESIDENTS AND INTERNS CHANGE (JUNE OR JULY AT MOST HOSPITALS)

As soon as you have decided to have surgery, check with your surgeon or the hospital and find out when their residents and interns change. If it turns out your surgery is scheduled near or at the time residents change—usually June or July—it is advisable to ask your surgeon to schedule your surgery either before or after the change occurs. We recommend this because things are hectic for new residents and interns. They must learn the ropes—where things are, what to do, and how to follow the orders of the attending doctors. Give them a chance to learn their jobs before you enter and become a patient. This will help you to avoid being a guinea pig or teaching vehicle. Ask your surgeon to schedule your surgery at least a month before the change or a month after the change occurs. And do not wait to make this request. This will help to plan ahead and avoid irritating your surgeon.

But suppose your surgeon responds to your request by telling you, "Look—it is very important for new residents and interns, who arrive in July each year, to gain experience. How can they do so if all the patients want to wait until August for their surgeries?"

We suggest that you reply by telling your surgeon, "Let the new doctors practice on someone else—not me." And you might also reassure your surgeon that very few patients will make such a request, so the new residents and interns will have many other patients on whom they can practice and learn the ropes.

RULE 40. ASK YOUR SURGEON TO VERIFY THAT YOUR ANESTHESIOLOGIST IS A BOARD-CERTIFIED MD

The anesthesiologist is important. He or she will control your lungs and breathing status while you are unconscious during surgery. It is essential the anesthesiologist be board certified, since this assures you that a reliable professional organization, the American Board of Anesthesiology, has examined qualifications and ability before granting certification. Remember that in some hospitals, anesthesiologists are permitted to practice who are either not board-certified MDs or who are nurse practitioners (NPs, not MDs). We do not mean to suggest that a nurse practitioner is not qualified to be an anesthesiologist. But it is too difficult for you, as a patient, to make such decisions: Do I need an MD anesthesiologist? Is a nurse practitioner sufficient? Play it safe and ask your surgeon to insist on an MD who is board certified in anesthesiology. Your surgeon has the authority to make this request.

RULE 41. ATTEMPT TO HAVE YOUR SURGERY IN A FULL-SERVICE HOSPITAL

The reasons why a full-service hospital is preferred are summarized in Appendix B, which explains why such hospitals are far more competent in handling emergencies that can occur with any surgical procedure. Selection of a hospital for surgery is usually done by the surgeon who will perform the surgery, not your doctor who has referred you to the surgeon. Therefore, the best way to follow this "full-service hospital" rule is to ask your doctor, when surgery is first discussed or considered, "Can you refer me to a surgeon who will operate at a *full-service* hospital that will permit me to have someone in my room at all times?" (And explain your 24/7 advocate request.) If this can't be done, or if, for any other reason, you find that your surgery will be performed at a second-

or third-tier hospital, you have an alternative: If you wish, elective surgeries allow you the time to locate a different surgeon who will do your surgery—as requested—at a full-service hospital. If your referring doctor is unable or unwilling to refer you to a surgeon who will operate using a full-service hospital, it is a simple matter to telephone a full-service hospital for help. Most of such hospitals have their own organized medical groups with well-qualified medical and surgical specialists of all types. Hopefully, your own doctor can then assist you to select one of these surgeons. Or, if you prefer, you may select one of these specialists without help from your doctor (see Rule 44).

On the other hand, you may wish to remain with a particular surgeon who operates at a lesser hospital and not push for a full-service hospital. This may be your best course of action. Certainly, a very competent surgeon in whom you have full confidence is the most important consideration even if he or she operates at a second-tier hospital.

To state it differently, selection of a competent surgeon is far more important than hospital selection, if you are required to make such a choice.

RULE 42. ARRANGE TO HAVE AN ADVOCATE/FRIEND REMAIN IN YOUR HOSPITAL ROOM WHEN NEEDED

At first blush, this may seem to be a peculiar rule. You may legitimately ask, "When I go into the hospital, why should I need any 'extra' person, like a friend/advocate, in the room with me? Aren't the nurses and doctors at the hospital always available very quickly if you press a button on your room device? And if it is a full-service hospital, aren't there also residents and interns available, as well as a hospitalist?" (See Rule 56 for a definition of *hospitalist*.)

Our answer: In an ideal hospital world, you would be absolutely right, but we don't live in such a world. Just remember: as we discussed in our introduction, things can go very, very wrong at any time, particularly between 10 p.m. and 6 a.m. Here is an example that explains what can happen if you don't have help when needed (we will call this person your "advocate").

You are in the hospital. You had serious surgery earlier in the day. It's 3 a.m. Suddenly, you find you are having serious difficulty in breathing. You press your call button and no one responds. You are alone. You are weak. The protective side rails are in place to prevent you from falling out of bed, and you do not know how to manipulate the release mechanism. You are in deep trouble.

But now let's assume you have followed this "advocate" rule. You call your advocate who is asleep in the chair or bed supplied by the hospital. You tell your advocate, "Please, get some help." He or she can immediately summon, by telephone or other means, the FIRST (Family Initiated Rapid Support Team; see Rule 51). Or your advocate can rush to the nearest nursing station.

There are many other important tasks that can be performed by your advocate, apart from the dramatic action just outlined:

- obtaining a drink of water or other fluids
- obtaining an extra blanket, newspapers, or other materials
- helping you to the bathroom
- helping to check if medications are for you (and not some-one else—Rule 72)
- reminding the nursing staff to bring your lunch
- reminding you to tell your doctor, when he or she arrives, about important new symptoms (it is easy to forget when you are sick and weak)

Of course, this rule should be used reasonably: If you are in full possession of your faculties and are mobile, you may not need such help. But if you have had a serious operation, such as heart surgery, and are weak and debilitated, such help may be essential 24/7. Or if you are in better shape but still weak (and concerned), you might find that help during daylight hours is sufficient.

This rule can be observed only if you enter a hospital that will permit an advocate to remain with you. (Some hospitals will allow this and some will not.) We also suggest that as soon as you know the identity of your hospital, you should call and verify that the advocate will be allowed for the time you require.

But what do you do if your doctor tells you, "Well, the hospital where I operate will not permit you to have such help. All visitors must leave by 8 p.m."? Then you must make a decision. Will you remain as this doctor's patient and enter a hospital where you are not permitted to have an advocate? Or will you find a different doctor who utilizes a hospital that will permit the advocate?

If you have found a surgeon in whom you (and your referring doctor) have confidence, you may decide to disregard this rule, since the choice of surgeon is clearly the most important consideration. If you do make such a decision, you should take comfort that our other rules will help to protect you even if you are not able to have an advocate in your room (see Rule 51 discussing the hospital kit and Rules 62 to 82 covering the entire period of hospitalization).

This recommendation for an advocate may take time to arrange. It may not be easy to find someone you can trust who is willing to give you the time required—which could be a week or two out of their life (depending upon your length of hospitalization and your medical problems). So, start to work on this project as soon as possible—you may need a month—or more. Of course, finding such an advocate may be a much simpler task if he or she is a spouse, relative, or other family member.

When you do locate a prospective advocate, be sure to explain the duties that your advocate will be expected to perform, particularly if there will be a time—perhaps hours or days—when you may be either unconscious, semiconscious, incoherent, or otherwise unable to handle all contingencies that may arise.

It is advisable to explain—and show—your hospital kit (Rule 51) to your advocate. Your kit contains information on whom to contact and what to do if an emergency occurs. It will give you valuable peace of mind to know that your advocate is not only willing to help you, but also has been properly prepared so he or she will be able to fulfill the duties discussed.

Finally, when you begin your hospital stay, starting with the day and time of entry, introduce your advocate to hospital personnel, including your doctors. Be careful that you structure this introduction to be positive and non-threatening: "I'd like to introduce my wife (or my friend). She has kindly agreed to stay with me in my room to help me. Perhaps she can also help the doctors and nurses and other hospital personnel if they request help."

Your advocate should always be friendly and positive, and should avoid any show of hostility or anger; your conduct should be the same (see Rule 4).

RULE 43. CONSIDER A SURGEON WHO IS SKILLED IN A PARTICULAR SURGERY, EVEN THOUGH HE OR SHE HAS A REPUTATION FOR POOR AFTERCARE

There are some highly competent surgeons who elect to perform such a large volume of operations that they cannot (or will not) perform the personal follow-up care that patients expect and need. They simply delegate such aftercare to their junior assistants and go on to their next surgery. Of course, you as a patient have the right to know if there will be no personal aftercare, and this may be a price that you are willing to pay to obtain your surgery from such a talented physician.

But before you agree to surgery by someone with this reputation, we suggest you ask your surgeon, "If I have serious complications after the surgery, who will see me and handle the problems?" Hopefully, your surgeon will reassure you that he or she will arrange for competent associates who will be available for all postoperative care. But if your surgeon is not willing to provide such reassurance, we suggest that you find another surgeon.

RULE 44. SELECT YOUR SURGEON CAREFULLY: INVESTIGATE, INTERVIEW, AND DECIDE

Now that we have considered the general rules to follow before selecting a surgeon, we will discuss how to apply and utilize these rules as you go through the selection process to achieve the best possible surgical result. You start the process by selecting a competent and experienced surgeon. "Competence" means the surgeon has been well trained and is skilled and adept. "Experience" means that he or she has performed your surgery many times—at least one hundred or more. But, as explained in the preceding eight rules (36–43), you must also consider other factors. Admittedly, these are less important than competence or experience, but you must keep them in mind. We are referring to rules such as the Monday-Tuesday-Wednesday rule (38), the full-service hospital rule (41), and the advocate rule (42).

As you approach the task of finding your surgeon, we suggest you begin by asking for a referral, from your own physician, to a physician he or she trusts and who has performed at least one hundred of the same type of surgery.

We do not advise that you suggest to your doctor a specialist that you "had heard of"—perhaps a doctor who is head of the surgical department of a well-known hospital. As a layperson, you have no way of knowing if a head of department is a competent surgeon or is simply one with political connections. In short, we suggest you begin your search by asking your own doctor. Hopefully, your own (trusted) doctor will refer you to a surgeon who he or she knows is competent, someone in whom your doctor has confidence based on experience. If for some reason you cannot obtain a referral from your doctor, consider obtaining a referral from one of the large medical groups that are affiliated with most major hospitals connected with university medical schools. More and more in recent years, large hospitals have established large and competent groups of doctors covering every medical specialty. It is a simple matter to make a telephone call to one of these respected institutions and ask them to refer you to a competent surgeon who has performed hundreds of the surgery that is involved.

But regardless of the method used to locate a prospective surgeon, before you make an appointment, do your own independent investigation:

1. Do a quick computer search or have a computer-savvy friend do it for you. Simply insert the doctor's full name, city, and state in the search bar. Example: "Laura Thurston, MD, Omaha, Nebraska." More and more MDs have extensive and very informative websites with much available information.

2. Do a search of your state's medical website. All fifty states license MDs and provide extensive information about the doctor's specialty, board certification, disciplinary record, lawsuits, and other information.

3. If you know or can locate someone who is acquainted with doctors or nurses, including OR nurses, ask them, "I am considering having Dr. X do my hip surgery. Can you tell me about his reputation as a surgeon? Is he considered competent?" (We realize this kind of inquiry may be impractical for many readers, but it is worth a try if you have the connections.)

After you have completed the steps just mentioned, it is time to call and make your first appointment with the surgeon. When you first call, verify that the surgeon will accept your insurance (see Rule 98). Once you have made the appointment, prepare. It is not complicated. Simply review Rules 36 to 43, which are the most important that apply when selecting a surgeon. If you are worried about remembering these eight rules, write yourself a brief reminder note. Do not bring in pages of notes, which would probably irritate the doctor. Also, do not begin speaking when you first sit down with the doctor. Let your new doctor take the lead, ask questions, and perform an examination if he or she wishes to do so.

At some point in your interview, perhaps after the doctor's examination or at some point that seems proper, be sure to say to the doctor—and try to pick the time diplomatically—"I have a few questions to ask. It won't take much time."

"First, I was told that you do this kind of surgery regularly and that you have done it hundreds of times. Is that correct?"

Experienced surgeons welcome such questions. If the doctor seems annoyed when you ask, it is definitely a warning sign. He or she may not have had the experience you want. Whoever referred you may not be aware of such lack of experience, but such experience is a very basic requirement.

Then, continue with the interview. Have in your hand your notes about Rules 36–43. Don't rush through these questions but don't dawdle. In other words, be *cool* and ask:

1. Will you personally do the surgery? I want to be sure that you do it and not simply supervise other student doctors who perform the surgery and hold the instruments. (Rule 36)
2. Will you be available for at least a week postoperatively if anything goes wrong? (Rule 37)
3. Can you do the surgery on a Monday, Tuesday, or Wednesday? (Rule 38)
4. Can we avoid June or July, or whenever the residents and interns change at the particular hospital you will be using? (Rule 39)
5. Will you be using a board-certified MD anesthesiologist? (Rule 40)
6. Will this be done at a full-service hospital with a functioning ICU, if necessary? (Rule 41)
7. Will this be done at a hospital that will permit me to have some friend or relative (advocate) stay with me—even overnight—when I am "out of it" or otherwise not able to communicate? (Rule 42)

During the entire time you are talking to the doctor, listen carefully and watch him or her closely. Is the doctor friendly? Is he or she relaxed or annoyed and bristling at your questions? Also, watch his or her hands. Do the hands tremble? Remember, sharp instruments will be held during the surgery only a few inches from your vital organs. You do not want a surgeon whose hands tremble. Don't hesitate to take the time you feel is needed to ask questions.

Don't worry if you conclude that the surgeon is unsatisfactory for any reason. Just keep in mind the fact that you will almost always have satisfactory alternatives (other doctors) if you have to look elsewhere. Most of our large and medium metropolitan areas have many satisfactory alternatives.

At the end of the interview exam, if you are comfortable with the doctor's answers, ask for the doctor to move ahead with the process of scheduling your surgery.

But let's assume that you are not comfortable with the doctor's answers. Examples:

- The surgery will be performed on a Thursday or a Friday.
- The doctor will not do the surgery herself, but will "carefully" supervise her residents or fellows who will be handling the operative instruments.
- The surgery will be done at a second- or third-tier hospital (see Appendix B).
- The hospital will not allow an advocate to stay in the room.
- The anesthesiologist will be a nurse practitioner, not a board-certified anesthesiologist MD.

If problems like the above exist, and if you have other choices in your community, you do have the option to tell the doctor that you are "not going to schedule surgery now," and will "sleep on the matter for a few days."

To help you make a decision (if you are uncomfortable with the surgeon's answers), look at the example of Jeptha:

Jeptha, age 38, required a hysterectomy. She was very glad to find Dr. Bob, to whom she had been referred by her internist. She felt confident after her interview, except for one item: Dr. Bob explained that he did all of his surgeries on Thursdays or Fridays. Of course, if Jeptha agreed to this, she would be violating Rule 38 (the Monday-Tuesday-Wednesday surgery rule). She told Dr. Bob about her concern. Dr. Bob assured her that he would be person-ally available at all times, but if for any reason he was not available, he would have her cared for by a thoroughly qualified doctor who would handle any emergency. Jeptha felt reassured and agreed to have Dr. Bob perform the surgery.

Jeptha made a wise decision despite the fact that she will be violating the Monday-Tuesday-Wednesday rule. The rule that fol-lows (Rule 45) explains, in more detail, how patients might consid-er and handle the problem of rule violations.

RULE 45. DON'T PANIC IF YOU MUST VIOLATE SOME OF RULES 36–43

We recognize that circumstances may make it impractical or even inadvisable to follow Rules 36–43. The previous example of Jeptha covered a violation of the Monday-Tuesday-Wednesday surgery rule. But now let's assume that the surgeon under consideration will operate at a second-tier hospital (see Appendix B) that may not have specialists readily available. We will use the example of Sarah:

Sarah had a tumor growing in her abdomen. Her oncologist had determined by a needle biopsy that it was not cancerous, but he told Sarah that it had to be removed, although there was no emergency. He recommended a general surgeon—Dr. Paul—in whom, he assured Sarah, he had "great confidence."

"He has done thousands of this type of surgery, and he is very good," he said.

Sarah liked Dr. Paul and asked, "Will the surgery be done at a full-service hospital?" Dr. Paul explained to Sarah that he per-formed his surgeries at a small neighborhood hospital close to his office, where he could easily take prompt care of his hospital patients.

This worried Sarah, who realized there might be a problem. She told Dr. Paul, "Suppose things go wrong and I need to see a specialist? There may not be any available at this hospital if a specialist is needed on short notice."

Dr. Paul was amused. "You're a real worry wart, aren't you?" he said. "But I like it. It tells me you want to have a successful surgery, and I agree with you absolutely. But relax. I have good friends in every specialty, and they are the best and will be available if needed; don't worry. I can bring them in any time they are needed, day or night—24/7."

Of course, not every doctor would be as reassuring and responsible as Dr. Paul. But Sarah's example, like that of Jeptha discussed previously, explains that rule violations can (under some circumstances) be handled.

Unlike the Jeptha and Sarah examples, what if you as the patient are simply not comfortable with the doctor's answers? What if you do not have a doctor as reassuring as Dr. Bob or Dr. Paul? You do have other choices—as discussed in Rule 44. However, starting the investigation and selection process all over again can be burdensome. The practical answer is to avoid the problems altogether. This can be done when surgery is first considered by asking your doctor or other referral source to refer you to a competent surgeon who performs surgery at a full-service hospital that also permits 24/7 advocates to remain in the room of their patients if such help is needed.

Now you can better understand why we suggest that you consider subjects like the need for an advocate (Rule 42) and a full-service hospital (Rule 41) when surgery is first discussed. Since all these rules involve elective or non-emergency surgery, the patient has ample time to think and decide: "Should I remain with a surgeon who will cause me to violate some important rules?" Or, "Since there is no need to rush into surgery, should I take the time to find another surgeon who will allow me to follow these 'full-service,' 'advocate,' and other rules?"

Rules to Observe after Selecting Your Surgeon

The following rules (46–50) contain some important dos and don'ts as you approach your date of surgery. They support the purpose of this section: to achieve the best possible result of your hospitalization and surgery. These rules involve matters within your general control as a patient, but they also require your doctor's consent and cooperation. You should try to observe these rules unless you have good reasons not to do so.

RULE 46. LET YOUR SURGEON SELECT HIS OR HER OWN METHOD AND INSTRUMENTS OF SURGERY

This is a time when you should listen carefully and trust your surgeon. If the surgeon wishes to make a large open incision, follow this advice. Or if the surgeon prefers to use a robotic device, allow him or her to do so. Do not ask the surgeon to use a certain method or device. There is a good reason for this admonition. Every surgeon has their own personal preference. Some will do a surgery with a special robotic device (the da Vinci Surgical System is one of them). Others do not like such devices, but may use them occasionally. If you ask the surgeon to use a particular method or device (which the surgeon does not usually use), the surgeon may agree to do so in order to placate you as the patient, but this request could be detrimental to your health. Why? Because the surgeon may have seldom used the requested method or device and is less adept as compared with the method usually used (many hundreds of times).

Every authority agrees: the important factor in surgery is the surgeon personally and not the device or technique used. So, don't play doctor. Allow your surgeon to select his or her own method or device.

Do not interpret this rule to mean you can't ask questions. On the contrary, if you wish to do so, you should not hesitate to ask questions. Here are a few:

- How will you do the surgery?
- How big will the incision be? (Two inches? Ten inches?)
- Will it be visible after a few months?
- Can you explain the possible major risks—if any?

RULE 47. ASK YOUR SURGEON IF HE OR SHE WILL USE A GENERAL OR A LOCAL ANESTHETIC AND WHETHER YOU HAVE A CHOICE

If a general anesthetic is used, you will be "out," which means you will be fully asleep and unaware of anything that occurs. If a local anesthetic is used, you will be awake—even if somewhat sedated—and aware of much of what is occurring even if your eyes are covered. It can be interesting; sometimes it can even be frightening—and some of us scare more easily than others. But if you have the stomach for it, and your surgeon allows you this option, we suggest that you seriously consider having a local rather than a general anesthetic. It is well known that if you don't go to sleep, you are better able to protect yourself. The following example explains this rule.

Sam entered the hospital for surgery on his left leg. He was not sure exactly why the surgery was needed, but he trusted his doctor and decided to have the surgery. His doctor said that either a local or a general anesthetic could be used and that Sam could choose: "You can have either one, and I've discussed this with the anesthesiologist, who agrees. There will be some pain, but it won't be bad, and if you want to, I think you could stand it easily."

Sam chose a local anesthetic. When Sam was in the operating room, before the surgery began, he noticed that the operating room personnel had covered up his left leg (where he thought the surgery was supposed to be done) and were doing something to his right leg—they were cleaning it with some kind of swab and shaving it. He asked the nurse and others in the operating room, "Why are you touching and working on my right leg? My surgery was supposed to be on my left leg." The nurse who was working on his leg blushed a deep red and apologized and quickly switched attention of the operating room personnel to prepare his left leg for surgery.

The point is obvious: Sam's choice of a local anesthetic prevented a major surgical error. Had Sam chosen a general anesthetic, tragedy may have resulted.

Note: Errors like that involving Sam are illustrations of the *preventable errors* discussed in our introduction.

RULE 48. DO NOT HAVE SURGERY ON A HOLIDAY OR WEEKEND

Holidays—either religious or secular—and weekends are the worst times to have any kind of surgery, major or minor. Often the primary surgeon who performed the surgery will not be available on weekends or holidays, and specialists are also much more difficult to obtain on a Saturday, Sunday, or holiday. Probably the worst time for surgery is between Christmas and New Year's Day, or during the entire Christmas season. The general idea is to avoid being relegated to the on-call doctors (who may not be familiar with your medical problem and the surgery performed). This is another reason to observe our Monday-Tuesday-Wednesday rule unless those days happen to coincide with a holiday.

Here is an example that illustrates this holiday/weekend rule:

Rudy, age 25, was told he needed gall bladder surgery. It was not an emergency situation, but he was told to schedule it within the next couple of weeks. This happened during the Christmas season, so Rudy scheduled his surgery for December 26, the day after Christmas, thinking to himself, "This will give me about a week during the holiday season to have the surgery and recuperate so I can go back to work on January 3 and not miss time from work."

The surgery was done on December 26, which was a weekday, and it went uneventfully. His surgeon told Rudy on the afternoon of the surgery, "Everything looks great. I'm leaving on a long-planned vacation for ten days, but you'll be fine. But if there is a problem, Dr. X, my associate, will take over and handle anything that comes up." His doctor waved goodbye and left.

The next morning, Rudy felt ill and his temperature was up to 104 degrees. The resident told him, "You have an infection; we want to call in a specialist in infectious diseases." Rudy waited until 6 p.m. that day, and then he called the nurse and said, "I'm supposed to see an infectious disease specialist because of my fever and the infection I was told I had. Where is the doctor?" The nurse said, "I don't know, but I'll look into it."

Rudy's example illustrates the dangers of holiday-time surgery. December 27, the day the fever developed, is the classic time you don't want to be in a hospital and have trouble. It is between Christmas and New Year's Day when almost everyone has plans. This is one of our more important rules!

RULE 49. BE CAREFUL ABOUT SCHEDULING SURGERY ONLY "TO AVOID LOSING TIME FROM WORK" IF SUCH SCHEDULING VIOLATES OTHER RULES

It is a very big mistake to let your job dictate when you have your surgery unless you can do so without violating the other rules. For example, if you have a two-week vacation scheduled, that can be an ideal time to have surgery providing you can have the surgery as we discussed in our other rules (on a Monday, Tuesday, or Wednesday, etc.). But do not allow work considerations to convince you to have elective surgery on a holiday or weekend. It is much too risky.

RULE 50. LET YOUR SURGEON DECIDE ON THE NUMBER OF SURGERIES THAT WILL BE PERFORMED

When patients are in the hospital for surgery, some might be tempted to ask their surgeon to do more than was originally planned: "Well, since I am having a facelift, why not also fix my heavy eyelids at the same time instead of having to come back for future surgeries?"

We advise readers to be very cautious before making this kind of request because your surgeon, wishing to be cooperative, may feel pushed into doing more surgery than is medically advisable. You should remain in your role as patient and let your doctor decide how many surgeries should be performed at one time. Remember: All surgeries have risks (see Rule 33), and more surgeries at the same time may mean more risks.

Caveat: Do not interpret this rule as a blanket cautionary warning against more than one surgery at a time. Your surgeon may have very good reasons for doing two or more surgical procedures while you are under the same anesthetic. But let your surgeon make such a decision. Do not urge him or her to do more than is advisable. The example of Isha explains:

Isha, age 30, had always wanted to fix her nose. It was long, curved, and very unsightly, and she felt she would look much better and be much happier if it was fixed. After careful inquiry, she located Dr. Jack, who had an excellent reputation and had obtained very good results with nose surgery on two of her friends. A date was agreed upon for the surgery.

Three weeks before surgery, Isha spoke to Dr. Jack, "You know, Dr. Jack, I've been thinking—while I'm having my nose job, how about fixing my eyelids also? They are very heavy-looking, and my girlfriends said I should ask you if perhaps you could fix them while I'm already in the hospital and getting surgery on my nose. What do you think?"

Dr. Jack responded, "I do not think this is wise. I know some plastic surgeons might disagree, and it is true that it will cost more money and take more time for a second hospitalization to come back later and fix your eyelids. But I am a very cautious guy, and I have seen other surgeons have big trouble when more than one surgery is done at a time. There is more risk of infection, more surgical trauma to your body, and other problems. Let's take care of your problems carefully—one at a time."

This is good advice and Isha should listen!

3

RULES COVERING THE LAST FEW WEEKS BEFORE PLANNED SURGERY

Rules 51–61

For all non-emergency surgeries, whether it is elective or even mandatory, you usually have some time to think and plan. You may have months or longer with purely elective surgery. But if the surgery is mandatory—for cancer or some other disease where time is a factor—you may have only days or weeks. But whatever time you do have should be used to prepare for this important life event.

The rules that follow will help you prepare for a successful hospitalization and surgery, and put you in the best position for recovery and discharge.

RULE 51. DURING THE WEEKS BEFORE HOSPITAL ENTRY, PREPARE, ASSEMBLE, AND LEARN HOW TO USE YOUR "HOSPITAL KIT"

You will have much on your plate in the weeks and days before hospital entry. These include both personal and business arrangements—particularly if your hospital and post-hospital period is extensive. But we urge you to remain focused on a primary goal: to both survive your surgery and hospitalization and emerge with a successful result. Your "hospital kit," which you should bring with you to the hospital, can play a very significant role in achieving such success. This kit will provide valuable protection if unforeseen events occur when you are ill and perhaps hardly conscious. Following is a description of the contents of the kit, along with explanations about using each item. Remember: this kit and its contents are not something you can simply buy pre-assembled. It must be personalized by you and for you. But not to worry! It is not difficult to put this kit together. Here is how you do it.

Preparing a Hospital Kit

This kit need not be large. You will need approximately the space provided by a small box—perhaps 9 × 12 × 1½ inches. Consider a small briefcase, a tote bag, or a separate container that can be placed in a large handbag. We do not think it is a good idea to allow items to float freely around inside the typical female handbag because its items can easily be lost, "buried," or misplaced.

The Contents of the Kit and How to Use Them

Important Telephone Numbers

Record these numbers on either 3 × 5 index cards or any 8½ × 11 copy paper. Remember that these are numbers of persons you can call if there is no response to your call device and if there is no other way to ask for help (from your advocate, a visitor, or some passing hospital employee). Be sure to do this before you enter the hospital. Be sure to record cell as well as landline numbers for the following people:

- Your spouse, companion, or significant other
- A parent or relative (mother, father, brother, sister)

- Anyone else you can depend on and can call 24/7
- Your advocate (Rule 42) if the advocate does not remain with you in your hospital room
- The hospital "FIRST" (Family Initiated Rapid Support Team). Many hospitals now have such teams who can be called as soon as problems occur—well before an alarm or monitor goes off—if "something does not feel right."
- Your primary care or concierge doctor (see Rule 100) who may have referred you to the surgeon or other specialist who is caring for you in the hospital
- The surgeon or other specialist in charge of your hospital stay
- 911—but before you call 911, use your whistle (see below), since 911 is the absolute *last* resort

All of the numbers mentioned above should be recorded and placed in your kit well before you enter the hospital. For readers who are especially energetic or compulsive, other telephone numbers can be added to the above, but these numbers will be difficult to obtain until after you enter the hospital. Readers should not feel that they must obtain these numbers, but for those who wish to do so, here are some additional numbers:

- The hospitalist (see Rule 56). Be sure that you obtain the full name of this MD so you are able to ask for him or her and not simply "the hospitalist."
- The chief of the hospital nursing staff. This is the head of all nurses in the hospital and would be the logical person to call if the nursing staff is not fulfilling their essential job of responding promptly to patients covered by their nursing station.
- The chief of the medical staff. This is the MD in charge of all doctors. He or she is an important person, and if you reach this person—who will be surprised by your call—it should certainly help to obtain action.

- The chief resident's office. This is the MD in charge of all residents, the trainees who often carry out a large percentage of the essential work at the hospital.

We do not believe that many of our readers will bother to obtain the telephone numbers of this latter group, but for the conscientious or especially interested readers, this is certainly an option.

We emphasize the need to obtain cell as well as landline numbers. This will double your chances of reaching the person you are attempting to contact.

Your Cell Phone/Smartphone and Charger

We suggest that you keep your portable phone (cell or smart) under your pillow or in some other convenient place where it is less likely to become lost. It is certainly advisable, particularly if you are out of your room, not to leave your telephone out in the open. You may go to the bathroom in your room or you may be out of your room for some tests, such as an X-ray, CT scan, or MRI. You probably will not take your telephone with you, so simply take reasonable steps to have it out of sight.

Hospital Kit Checklist

☐ Important phone numbers
☐ Phone and charger
☐ Extra reading glasses
☐ Whistle
☐ Medications
☐ Spiral-bound note pad
☐ $10 cash
☐ Photo ID
☐ Two permanent black markers and pens
☐ Small LED flashlight
☐ Transparent tape
☐ Dental floss

Extra Reading Glasses

Of course, this assumes that you need glasses for reading, and if you do, glasses are easy to lose, so the extra pair will come in handy.

A Small, Loud Whistle

You may wonder "why would I even need a whistle in the hospital?" Answer: An emergency can occur at any time of the day or night. You may need help immediately for some emergency. If there is no response to your call device and if there is no other method that can be used to call for help (your advocate, a visitor, a passing employee), then your whistle may be the only immediate method of obtaining help when you need it. These whistles are readily available at hardware or other stores, such as Target, Walmart, and many other retail establishments. A whistle—at least the one you should be purchasing—will be easy to hear even through a solidly closed hospital door. Be sure you try the whistle so you know it is loud and piercing. In addition to the whistle mentioned (which does take some effort to blow), some readers might also consider adding an electric whistle or horn. This requires no physical effort (if you are sick, tired, weak, and desperate), except pressing a button. These air/horn whistles may be a bit more difficult to locate, but all you need do is go to your search engine (Google, etc.) and put in "air whistle" or "air horn" and you will be inundated with information about where and how you buy one.

Medications

Many of our readers are already taking medications, perhaps two, three, five, or even ten per day. Most readers will be using the ubiquitous seven-day plastic container, and of course you should take sufficient meds to cover what you think will be the length of your hospital stay. But it is important, per Rule 59, to first obtain the permission of your doctor, who will need to have hospital consent to allow you to take and use such medications.

A Small 6 × 9 Spiral Pad

We suggest a spiral binding to avoid loss of notes. Of course, we do not feel you need turn yourself into a daily diary writer; in fact, you should not feel compelled to keep a diary. But there are times when you should be making notes. For example, you may sustain some injury in the hospital, such as falling out of bed and injuring your head. Since this might lead to a serious problem, we suggest you make a detailed written note of such an incident, by noting the date and time as well as a detailed description, per Rule 102. If you are too sick or otherwise unable to write, try to have the note made by your advocate or any cooperative visitor. Such notes can (later) be placed in your medical file per Rule 25.

Less Than $10 in Cash

No need to risk losing any more money.

Your Photo ID

We suggest you make a photocopy of your driver's license and leave the original home. Insofar as credit cards are concerned, these are optional items, but you might need to make purchases in the hospital; they are handy to have and can easily be replaced if necessary.

At Least Two Permanent Black Felt-Tip Markers and Two Ball Pens

You may need to mark your body if you have forgotten to do so per Rule 52. Or there may be some other reason why you may wish to make some type of note that is very easy to read by anyone. You may also need to create or refresh new signs or notes as discussed by Rules 52 and 66.

A Small LED Flashlight

These small flashlights are very easy to obtain in almost any pharmacy or hardware store. These LED flashlights are approximately the size of a pack of Lifesavers. Of course, it is rare for power to fail in a hospital, but why take a chance?

A Medium-Size Roll of Scotch Tape

We suggest you obtain the type upon which you can write with a ballpoint pen. This tape can be used as described in Rule 52.

Dental Floss

Dispensers are available at all pharmacies and any other stores that sell toothbrushes. Besides using it for your teeth, you can use it to create a necklace around your neck to hold your printed warning to doctors and hospital personnel to remind them about your allergy to medicines, your pacemaker, or anything (see Rule 52).

This hospital kit may cause some eyes to roll if the hospital staff or doctors discover it. So it is probably wise to be discreet and put the kit in a drawer or some other unobtrusive place.

RULE 52. A DAY OR TWO BEFORE HOSPITAL ENTRY, USE A PERMANENT BLACK FELT-TIP MARKER TO PRINT WARNINGS ABOUT ALLERGIES AND BODY SURGERY

Doctors and other hospital personnel must be notified and re-minded about two important facts. First, they need to be re-minded about the location of surgery on your body in order to prevent a mistake—e.g., surgery in the wrong location or on the wrong arm or leg. And second, they need to know about your allergies or other important facts that may influence your treatment or well-being—such as if you have a pacemaker, a stent, or other device.

1. Warning: Surgery on the Correct Part of the Body

Indicate what part of your body should and should not be the subject of surgery. Use your black permanent felt-tip marker from your hospital kit and block print on your body—in large capital letters—where the surgery should and should not take place. If there is to be surgery on the arm, print directly at the surgical location on the arm "surgery here." Do the same for surgery on all parts of the body. It is also advisable, if an arm or leg is involved, to print another warning on the other arm or leg: "not this leg," for example. To be sure that your warning will not be "accidentally" washed off, be sure that your marker has the word "permanent" on it.

2. Warning: Allergies or Items like a Pacemaker or Stent

If you are allergic to a medication, use your permanent black felt-tip marker and print a warning on any 8½ × 11-inch paper or poster stock. Do the same if you are allergic to penicillin. Print: "I am allergic to penicillin" or any other warning that is applicable (pacemaker, stent, etc.). Make at least three of these posters and use them as follows:

- Tape one to your bed—either the foot or the head of the bed—using the transparent tape from your hospital kit.
- Make a "necklace" using a second poster. Use string or dental floss taped to both sides of the poster and hang it around your neck so it sits on your chest and will be a warning to nurses and doctors and any other hospital personnel.
- Ask a nurse to place the third poster on the top cover of your chart (taped or otherwise fastened) so that it will be secure and very visible to whichever doctor, resident, intern, fellow, or nurse happens to pick up the chart.

RULE 53. EXCEPT FOR YOUR HOSPITAL KIT, LEAVE YOUR VALUABLES AT HOME TO PREVENT LOSS OR THEFT

There are many items you should leave at home when you go to the hospital. This includes anything you do not wish to lose (or have stolen). This includes jewelry, such as necklaces, wedding rings, bracelets, and earrings. Do not bring your medical file; it is valuable and irreplaceable. Of course, if you don't care about loss of such items, this rule is unnecessary.

RULE 54. IF YOU WILL HAVE A PRIVATE-DUTY NURSE, MAKE ARRANGEMENTS AT LEAST A WEEK BEFORE HOSPITAL ENTRY

It can take time to locate a qualified and compassionate private-duty nurse—RN or LVN. Your doctor or the hospital should be asked to help; they have the contacts and experience to do this. But remember this: private-duty nurses are expensive. The charge can exceed $500 for an eight-hour shift, and such expenses are usually not covered by insurance. But on the plus side, a private-duty nurse around the clock will probably eliminate the need for a 24/7 friend/relative/advocate (Rule 42). Or you may opt for a private-duty nurse during only one shift—perhaps 11 p.m. to 7 a.m.—and then utilize your advocate during the time the nurse is not present.

As a practical matter, most readers will probably not need this rule because they won't be able to afford the very large expense of a private-duty nurse—particularly if the private-duty nurse is employed for more than a day or two.

You might also consider arranging for a private-duty nurse for only the critical day or two after surgery when you are either "out of it" or very sick and unable to protect yourself or communicate; you may be unconscious or practically so for several days. But these are things you should discuss with your surgeon. The bottom line is to not wait for the day before surgery. Arrange for any such nurse—if you are going to have one—well ahead of time.

RULE 55. REVIEW HOSPITAL PAPERWORK SEVEN TO TEN DAYS BEFORE ENTRY

Becoming a hospital patient can be hectic and nerve-racking. It is better to take your time at home where you can read the many documents required by the hospital. Perhaps a friend or your 24/7 advocate (Rule 42), if you have found one, can help you.

You can either personally pick up the hospital paperwork or send someone else. Or you can request that they be mailed to you unless they are online and you can receive them as an attachment. Of course, this requires that you be computer savvy, so it may not be a practical suggestion.

Before putting your signature on any document, be sure to call the hospital and ask, "Should I bring in my documents with my signature on them?" Some hospitals require you to sign at the time of admission; it is easy to find out by a phone call.

Don't be concerned if the hospital refuses to give you the sign-in documents in advance. They may tell you, "We will handle the paperwork when you check in at the time of admission." Do not argue. Remember, be friendly!

Whenever and however you obtain the sign-in paperwork, whether in advance or at the time of hospital entry, the approach is the same:

1. Do not expect to understand much of what you read. With two exceptions, simply skim through and sign all of them as requested and don't worry or hassle. Don't be concerned that "I may be signing away valuable legal rights." And don't worry if your 24/7 advocate also admits that he or she is confused. To repeat: relax and sign (except for the two items next discussed).

2. Here are the two exceptions we want you to understand and handle. They involve your consent to surgery and credit card authorization. These two documents may be buried in your pile of other documents. Watch for them! We will discuss each separately:

Exception 1: The Surgical Consent (See Appendix C)

Look for the surgical consent. It may say "Consent to Surgery" or different words may be used. It gives the surgeon the right to operate on you. If you can't easily find it, ask someone at the hospital—either in person or by telephone—"Please tell me, where in your forms is the Consent to Surgery?" You must find it. When you do, alter it so that you are giving the right to do surgery only to your surgeon. Do not ask for "permission" to change the form. Quietly, and without saying anything to the hospital intake personnel, draw a line through the printed material that would allow your surgery to be performed by someone else. To help you understand this rule, we have included a sample consent showing our suggested alteration in Appendix C.

You need not be a lawyer to understand this rule. Just make sure that your surgical consent is corrected before you sign it, so that it gives the right to do surgery to your doctor and no one else. If you are not sure how to alter the form, or if you are otherwise confused, print the following words just above your signature: "I grant only Dr. [*name of your doctor*] permission to do this surgery."

Also, don't forget that there are various *backup rules* mentioned elsewhere in our book that require that you also have several personal discussions with your surgeon, during which the surgeon agrees that he or she will personally perform the surgery. If there is some question, you might mention you have heard that, particularly at major hospitals, the actual surgery is performed by residents, interns, or fellows to train them, and while you certainly think this is a good idea, "I do not want this to happen at my surgery."

We realize we have suggested you have this discussion with your surgeon several times, but our repetition is intentional. Memories—even for skillful surgeons—can be short, particularly in the hectic times leading up to the surgery itself. Therefore, better to be safe, not sorry!

Finally, do not worry if you do not find and alter the surgical permission document. Per these rules, you will be reminding your surgeon several different times of his obligation—and agreement—to personally perform the surgery.

Exception 2: Credit Card Authorization

Do not sign any credit card authorization or put your hospital bill or hospital obligation on a credit card. The reason for this is simple. Once your credit card company pays your bills, whether they are in the hundreds or thousands, it will be impossible to ever make a deal. You cannot do business with a credit card company. But if you enter a hospital and they require a deposit—say $500— you are far better off to write them a check if you can do so, or somehow pay them the deposit even if you borrow money from someone else. Or take any other reasonable means to avoid using a credit card. The reason is that once you give that credit card authorization, you are almost guaranteeing you will never be able to reduce the hospital bill or work out some arrangement to pay the bill within your budget. Also, this is a good reason why you should try to pick up the hospital entry documents—as we mentioned previously—seven to ten days in advance of hospitalization to take home and review with help, if possible, to make sure you are not signing any credit card authorization.

RULE 56. IN THE WEEKS BEFORE ENTRY, DETERMINE IF A HOSPITALIST WILL BE AVAILABLE TO SEE PATIENTS

Hospitalists are experienced physicians who are employed by some—but not all—hospitals to help with patient care if the regular attending doctor is not available. These special doctors are particularly important if a patient has an emergency medical problem, perhaps at odd hours when neither the regular or "covering" doctor is available. Such doctors can provide important care that may not be available from residents, interns, or other substitute doctors whose expertise is questionable.

RULE 57. IF YOU ARE ILL BEFORE YOUR ELECTIVE OR NON-EMERGENCY SURGERY, ASK YOUR DOCTOR ABOUT POSSIBLE CANCELLATION

It is usually a mistake to have surgery if you are sick. For example, if you have an infection, are coughing or sneezing, have some type of stomach flu, or are otherwise ill, notify your regular doctor and/ or surgeon as soon as you are aware of the problem. Remember, this is elective or non-emergency surgery, so why take the risk? It is generally smart to wait until you are in good physical shape before you have elective surgery. Of course, there may be times when the surgery should not be postponed, but this is a decision to be made by your doctor.

RULE 58. ASK YOUR DOCTOR WHICH MEDICATIONS YOU SHOULD BE TAKING OR DISCONTINUING BEFORE YOU ENTER THE HOSPITAL

Many patients take medication regularly—particularly older patients. For example, a patient may be diabetic, have prostate cancer, or have a cholesterol problem. Patients may be taking medications to handle all these problems. Be sure to ask your surgeon or your regular doctor about which medications you should continue taking and which you should stop. Most of the time, if you are facing surgery, the doctors will have you stop medications for a few days ahead of time—particularly aspirin. But it is not your role to make decisions about medicine. All that we suggest you do is talk to your doctor or surgeon and let them figure out what you should take and what you should stop taking before entering the hospital. Also, find out if you should avoid eating or drinking prior to entering the hospital, although this problem might be handled once you enter and before surgery takes place. Don't forget to ask about powders, perfumes, or creams. In any event, simply make it a habit to ask and make a note of what is said so you will be able to properly follow doctor's orders and protect yourself.

RULE 59. ASK YOUR DOCTOR'S PERMISSION TO BRING YOUR OWN MEDICATION TO THE HOSPITAL INSTEAD OF TAKING THOSE SUPPLIED BY THE HOSPITAL

Many patients are on medications for blood pressure, cholesterol, diabetes, and other conditions. The standard practice of hospitals is to tell you they will provide the medications while you are a patient. Usually, they do not want you to bring your own medication to the hospital. However, hospital personnel often make medication mistakes (see Rule 72). One way you can avoid being a victim of these errors is to use your own medications.

To avoid controversy with the hospital and to obtain their consent, make arrangements in advance so that you, your doctor, and the hospital are all in agreement about your bringing your own medications.

Also, using your own medication has some other positive consequences. You will not be charged large amounts of money for medications, and neither will your insurance carrier. So, both you and your insurance carrier, including Medicare, will benefit if you can avoid unnecessary charges for medication supplied by the hospital.

Of course, there may be good reason *not* to bring your own medication to the hospital (if you are too ill, incompetent, or otherwise disabled). This also should be discussed with your doctor before hospital entry.

RULE 60. WELL BEFORE SURGERY, ARRANGE FOR POSTOPERATIVE CARE

When surgery is first considered, you should discuss with your doctor the nature and extent of postoperative disability and what you are going to need in the way of help after the surgery. But if you have not had such a discussion, you still have time to do so in the weeks before your surgery. You may wish to ask the doctor to not send you home after the surgery, but to put you in some place that is a step between hospitalization and home—often called a *skilled nursing facility* or *rehab* or some other name. This may be necessary if there is no one at home to care for you. On the other hand, patients with financial means may arrange for someone to provide home care: cooking meals, handling household chores, and providing nursing care (if required). Attention should also be directed to children and spouse. Will they also need help during your postoperative period? It is important to make such arrangements before the surgery when you have the time and energy to do so.

RULE 61. VERIFY THAT YOU HAVE HAD A PREOPERATIVE PHYSICAL EXAMINATION

Every patient must have a *preoperative* physical examination. This is usually a few days ahead of time or perhaps the day before surgery. It is a simple matter to ask, diplomatically (if there is any question), "Have I had my preoperative physical?" Do not undergo surgery if you are told, for example, "Oh, that is not necessary." This is one time where you are in charge, and in view of the fact that this surgery is elective, don't take any chances. Mistakes can be made, and patients can undergo surgery who are simply not in physical shape to survive the surgery. We realize we are talking about a small percentage of patients, but a preoperative physical is essential for patient health and safety.

4

RULES DURING HOSPITALIZATION

Rules 62–82

Hospitalization (whether elective or not) for any period of time requires a new and different mindset on your part as the patient, as compared with the mindset you'd have for medical care outside of the hospital. Except for your advocate, if you have one (Rule 42), you will be entirely dependent upon the abilities and motivation of doctors and other hospital personnel, because you will be under their care and control 24/7. It is completely different from your familiar home surroundings, where you know what you should be doing to protect your health and general well-being: fixing meals, taking medicine, resting, and all other day-to-day activities. But during hospitalization, other people—strangers—now perform these functions. You are no longer in control. You are vulnerable, particularly while you are weak, less alert, perhaps mentally disordered, or unconscious. The rules in this chapter are designed to protect you from the dangers described in our introduction during your entire stay in the hospital. Study these rules carefully!

RULE 62. HAVE YOUR FRIEND/ADVOCATE HELP WITH THE CHECK-IN PROCEDURE

Rule 42 explains the need for and function of your advocate. It is definitely advisable to have this person present with you as you go through the check-in process and not wait until you are in your hospital room. During the check-in process, you may be nervous. You may not have yet signed the necessary documents (many patients will not have followed Rule 55 about obtaining hospital paperwork a week or two in advance). So, it will be comforting to have a friend/helper at your side as you are told to "sign here" or do something else. Or you may be asked confusing questions. Your advocate can help you scan through the voluminous paperwork so you can identify and deal with the two essential items discussed in Rule 55:

1. The surgical consent (which you will need to alter)
2. Credit card authorization (which you should not sign)

As far as other hospital documents are concerned, it is perfectly fine to ask what you are signing, but don't worry if you do not understand what they mean—even after asking questions.

Remember: Most of our rules are applicable only to elective and non-emergency surgery. Therefore, if you have any significant problems—financial or otherwise—as you are going through the entry process, you have the option to refuse to sign and to leave. (See Rule 33 and the cautions concerning elective surgery.)

RULE 63. BOTH YOU AND YOUR ADVOCATE SHOULD ALWAYS BE DIPLOMATIC, FRIENDLY, AND COOPERATIVE WITH EVERYONE AT THE HOSPITAL

From the moment you start the hospital check-in process until the moment you are discharged days or even weeks later, avoid whining, complaining, or otherwise creating a "problem." You and your advocate should be kind to all hospital personnel, including doctors, nurses, techs, and cleaning staff. If you remain pleasant and cooperative throughout your hospital stay, it is much more likely that your time in the hospital will be a positive experience. Furthermore, it is well to remember that as a hospital patient, you will be vulnerable at all times. Never forget that if anyone wishes to neglect, irritate, ignore, or injure you, you are vulnerable! Therefore, be sweet! If there is a provocation or reason to be irritated, try to turn the other cheek. Both you and your 24/7 advocate should go out of your way not to antagonize anyone.

If you do find it necessary to complain about anything—and such an occasion may certainly arise—try to do it carefully and diplomatically, and keep in mind the fact that retribution can be very easy, as indicated by the example of Frances that follows:

Frances was hospitalized because of high blood pressure. She did not have a 24/7 advocate. From the very beginning, she was a "difficult" patient. She complained about everything—the hospital was cold, there were not enough blankets, it was noisy. When she spoke to the nurses, her tone was demanding and critical.

When the tech arrived to administer very mild blood pressure medicine, Frances's reputation was already well known on the floor. She literally barked at the medical tech who was administering nitro paste, which he smeared on her body (a method of lowering blood pressure). She complained the paste was "irritating and cold." Nevertheless, the tech completed the paste application and left the room.

Several hours later, Frances suffered a stroke—possibly because the paste treatment lowered her blood pressure too quickly (this is a danger all blood pressure patients face). This stroke was a contributing factor to her death a few months later.

It was not clear just why Frances had the stroke; it may have occurred even without the "paste treatment." It was also possible that too much nitro paste was applied by the tech and was the cause of the stroke. But this example illustrates how Frances, by being friendly, could have avoided creating negative feelings toward her in the mind of the medical technician. Just remember the cautions discussed in the beginning explanation of this rule. Patients—like Frances in our example—are vulnerable.

RULE 64. CONFIRM THAT YOUR HOSPITAL WRISTBAND HAS YOUR CORRECT INFORMATION

Verify that your wristband has your correct name, date of birth, and hospital number. There is a good reason for this simple rule. Many patients have similar names. There are many Smiths, Joneses, Goldbergs, Martinezes, and so on. If your wristband has a mistake in either your name or date of birth, it can lead to disastrous medication and treatment errors (see Rule 72).

RULE 65. RIGHT AWAY, LEARN HOW TO WORK THE CALL DEVICE AND OTHER EQUIPMENT IN YOUR HOSPITAL ROOM

Hospital call devices, electric beds, and even TV sets can seem complicated. You and your 24/7 advocate should learn how to use them as soon as you are settled in your room. The call device is the most important. If there is any question, simply ask the nurse or other hospital personnel how it is to be used. Verify that you understand what to do before this person leaves your room. The most important item is how to call the nurse if there is a problem (can't breathe, bleeding, pain, etc.).

Other functions, such as how to use the bed controls and your TV set, are less important. But you should feel comfortable that you and your 24/7 advocate know how the various devices are to be used. Of course, this rule is even more important if you are alone and do not have a 24/7 advocate.

RULE 66. PROMPTLY AFTER ADMISSION, VERIFY THAT YOUR BODY WARNING SIGNS AND OTHER PRINTED SIGNS ARE PLACED AND VISIBLE

Rule 52 explains how you should compose warning signs for both your body and for placement in your hospital room. As soon as you are settled in your room, review this rule and follow through with verification of the following:

- Your body warning signs are clear, readable, and correct.
- Other warning signs are placed where they will be visible to the doctors and other hospital personnel.

RULE 67. BEFORE SURGERY, RECONFIRM YOUR SURGEON WILL BE THE ONE PERFORMING THE SURGERY

You may think that all you need do is tell your surgeon, per Rule 36, that you want him or her to be the surgeon and to wield the scalpel. But you must understand that at the major hospitals, which are usually affiliated with medical schools, there is a tremendous desire—and a very laudable one—to train residents and interns so they will be proficient in their craft. The point is that in the hectic times in an operating room—particularly if the doctor has a surgical schedule where he is going to do two or three in one day—it is easy for the most competent surgeon to simply forget a promise and to do "the usual," which is to supervise and have others, such as residents and fellows, actually perform the surgery. So there is nothing wrong with reminding the doctor, even two or three times, about the understanding that you are authorizing the surgery be done by him or her and by not any assistants. As you will see by the other rules in this book, we suggest that this request should be made several times: when surgery is first considered, when you enter the hospital, and even as you are being wheeled into the operating room (if you are conscious enough to talk). You can say *jokingly*, "I hope no one will be offended if I again confirm this surgery is going to be done by Dr. [*your doctor*] and not by some other doctor who is supervised by my doctor."

We realize this may sound like a belt and suspenders, but a large percentage of surgeries are done this way, and patients never know. Just don't let it happen to you.

RULE 68. BEFORE ENTERING THE OPERATING ROOM, CONFIRM WHICH ANESTHETIC WILL BE ADMINISTERED (LOCAL OR GENERAL)

Before you enter the hospital, you should know, after a discussion with your surgeon, whether you will be having a local or general anesthetic (Rule 47). It is also advisable to meet with the anesthesiologist before your surgery and before you start your hospitalization. If this meeting has not taken place before you enter the hospital, do so after entry.

At this meeting, you should mention any major health problems (asthma, COPD, emphysema, etc.) and confirm which anesthetic will be used. If, for any reason, such a meeting has not taken place, you should arrange to have a telephone discussion to cover these topics.

Finally, just in case someone "forgets," it does no harm—with a smile—to confirm the arrangement. Do this just before surgery, while you are still conscious. Ask your nurse or doctor, "As I understand it, I am going to have a local anesthetic," or "I'm going to have a general anesthetic." This will assure that there will be no last-minute hitches in the event the word has not gotten through to those in the operating room. This discussion can be had when you are actually in the operating room, providing you are still conscious. It is rare for such a misunderstanding to occur, but it definitely does happen.

RULE 69. PRIOR TO SURGERY, TELL YOUR SURGEON IF YOU HAVE REMOVABLE DENTURES, IMPLANTS, STENTS, OR SIMILAR ITEMS

Inquiry should have been made by either your surgeon or one of the doctors involved in your care before surgery. Remember that dentures can be dislodged and drop down into your throat when you under the anesthetic, and this can be very dangerous. Pacemakers may be affected by operating room procedures (use of electric instruments), and the same may be the case if you have stents or other hardware in your body. Problems are easily avoided by fully disclosing all such items to your surgeon in advance of surgery.

RULE 70. ASK YOUR DOCTOR: "WHAT OTHER DOCTOR WILL BE SEEING ME DURING MY HOSPITALIZATION?"

It is important and comforting to know which doctors, aside from your surgeon, will be seeing you while you are a hospital patient. For example, if you have had surgery and have a problem late at night (or during a weekend), your surgeon may arrange to have an associate who will be on call. Or your surgeon may call in consultants in various specialties such as neurology, gastroenterology, oncology, or others. Your doctor may suspect you have other problems, or he or she may simply wish to rule out other possibilities. But whatever the reason, you should inquire so you know your doctor's concerns and what other doctors will be requested to see you in the hospital. This might happen before surgery if your surgeon wished to have a cardiologist check your heart. Or after surgery, your surgeon might feel there is a possible infection, and then call in an infectious disease specialist. If you know the name and the specialty of the doctor who has been asked to see you, you would be able to tell your doctor whether or not this consultant has actually come to see you. Sometimes there may be a miscommunication, and the consultant(s) may not arrive as requested. If you have the name (or names), you will then be able to tell your doctor (or the nurse) that Consultant X has not yet been to see you.

You might also ask your surgeon if he or she will supply you with the telephone numbers—office or cell—of his or her associate, whom you can call if your surgeon is not available.

RULE 71. IN THE HOSPITAL, MAKE NOTES OF IMPORTANT EVENTS TO INCLUDE IN YOUR MEDICAL FILE

Things happen when you are in the hospital—whether for surgery, treatment, or observation. We do not suggest you spend your day writing about inconsequential items, but some events should be recorded when they happen (unless you are too sick to write). Your hospital kit (Rule 51) will supply you with writing materials.

This rule applies to matters that you should document in addition to the "negative" events discussed in Rules 102–104, which concern possible legal consequences (wrong medicine brought by a nurse or other negligent conduct). For example, suppose your entire right arm, from your shoulder to your fingertips, suddenly becomes numb, and you have no feeling whatsoever. Or suppose your eye, which just had surgery, suddenly loses vision. These are matters you should carefully record with date and time so they can be reported to your doctors. In addition, when you are discharged and return home, these dated notes should be kept in your medical file (Rule 25). They will help you to provide accurate and important history to your doctors in the future.

RULE 72. BEFORE TAKING ANY MEDICATION, VERIFY IT WAS PRESCRIBED FOR YOU AND NOT SOME OTHER PATIENT

This rule is based upon an unfortunate fact. Study after study throughout the United States for many years has revealed that 20 to 25 percent of all hospital medications that are administered are done so in error—either the wrong patient, the wrong medication, the wrong dose, or the wrong time. To avoid being the victim of such error, you as the patient, with the help of your 24/7 advocate if available, should take reasonable precautions.

Always ask questions before accepting either oral medication (pills, liquid, etc.) or injections, and ask the following questions (it doesn't matter which question is asked first):

1. "What is the name of the patient who is to take this medication?" Or, you could ask, "What's my name?" If the nurse or other person bringing the medication seems hostile or says, "Why are you asking?" simply reply, "I just want to avoid any possible mistake. Please answer my questions."
2. "What is the name of the medication?" If this question brings a hostile response, give the same response indicated for number 1 above.

The example of Elena explains this rule:

Elena, age 30, was in the hospital for observation and possible hysterectomy. At approximately ten o'clock in the morning, a member of the hospital staff—either a nurse's aide or a nurse (Elena was not sure)—came with her pills in a small container with a cup of water and asked Elena to please take her medication.

Elena asked her, "Well, what is in this medication?" The nurse said, "I believe it is something for blood pressure."

Elena knew she had no blood pressure problem because the doctor had said her blood pressure was fine, so she then next asked the nurse, "Well, what is my name?"

The nurse said, "Look, why are you asking me these questions? Please take the medication. I have other patients to do." She was irritated.

Elena persisted and said, "Well, what is the name of the patient who is supposed to take this? I'm asking because I didn't think I had a blood pressure problem."

The nurse acted a bit flustered, but she looked at the slip in her hand and said, "Your name is Mary Sperling, isn't it?"

Elena said, "No. You have the wrong patient." Quickly, the nurse said, "Oh, sorry about that," and left the room.

Some hospital personnel will probably be irritated by such questioning, but your health (and your very life) can be in jeopardy with the wrong medication. So *stick to your guns* and do not take medication if you are not satisfied with the answers you receive. (This may be the time to press your call device button and obtain answers from the on-duty RN.)

This rule does assume that you (or your advocate) have some knowledge of the medications you are supposed to be taking. This is why you should ask your doctor to keep you informed about each medication that is prescribed.

You should ask these questions even if your bed is equipped with a scanning device (Rule 73). These devices are very good, but they are not foolproof, so ask!

If the medication brought to your hospital room is in a hanging plastic bag (or bags) from which a tube hangs down, you or your advocate should also look to verify that it is your full name and correct date of birth. This will avoid the problem of the orderly or other technician bringing someone else's bag to your room.

RULE 73. IF YOUR ROOM HAS A BEDSIDE SCANNING DEVICE TO CHECK MEDICATION, MAKE SURE IT IS USED

Some hospitals have a medical scanning device next to the bed. It is programmed to verify that the patient is receiving the correct medication—that which was ordered by the physician. It is matched with the patient through a bar code so that when medication is brought into the room, the device makes sure that the bar code on the patient's device matches the bar code of the medication that is being delivered.

It is possible that your hospital does not have this device. But this should not raise any concern on your part. Simply follow through on the other rules to make sure the medication brought to you is ordered for you by your doctor (see Rule 72).

This rule is well illustrated by a famous example—that of twins who were born at a major hospital. They happened to be the children of a well-known Hollywood actor. Because of an error in medication, the twins were given a huge and dangerous dose of heparin and almost died. This type of tragedy could be avoided if there was a bedside scanning device, assuming it was working properly. It would be particularly important for newborns, young children, elderly patients, or anyone else who may be incapacitated or incompetent. Again, this underscores the value of an advocate (Rule 42) who can help protect the patient by watching and asking the questions explained in Rule 72 to verify that correct medication is given to the patient.

RULE 74. IF YOU HAVE A SERIOUS MEDICAL PROBLEM, INSIST ON BEING SEEN BY AN EXPERIENCED MD; DO NOT ALLOW A DELAY UNTIL YOUR TREATING DOCTOR OR SURGEON RETURNS

This rule applies to a situation when your regular treating doctor or surgeon is not available and cannot be contacted. It may occur on a Saturday or Sunday, in the evening, or in the early morning hours. There may be a serious change in your condition: difficulty in breathing, severe bleeding, or a sudden and different type of pain. You would definitely want to be seen by an experienced doctor if your own doctor is not available, either personally or by telephone. Sometimes—even in a full-service hospital—a nurse, intern, or resident may decide that you should "wait until Monday" or the following day, if the problem occurs during the week. Or the problem may occur on a Saturday or Sunday, and someone in the hospital—either a junior doctor or a nurse—may decide the problem can wait until your surgeon returns from a weekend out of town.

A delay like this can be a huge mistake. As far as you the patient are concerned, your best interest requires that you be seen by an experienced physician who is qualified to decide if immediate action is required or if it is safe and advisable to delay action until your treating doctor is available. After all, in a full-service hospital there are usually experienced doctors, including a hospitalist (Rule 56), who can be made available. Or perhaps your doctor has given you the name of his or her on-call associate (Rule 70) who is supposed to see you after hours if your doctor is not available. This would definitely be the time for you to call this doctor.

Again, the key concept: *Don't wait—act!*

RULE 75. IF YOU DISCOVER THAT DOCTORS OR OTHER HOSPITAL PERSONNEL DISAGREE WITH THE TREATMENT YOU ARE RECEIVING, INVESTIGATE AND CONSIDER A SECOND OPINION

Sometimes a patient who pays attention may overhear a nurse or someone else tell one of your doctors (out in the hall where they don't realize you are listening), "Doctor, I think you should stop this medication" or some similar criticism. It may be a conflict between a nurse and a junior doctor, resident, intern, or someone else. However, as soon as you are aware of such a conflict, we suggest that you contact your doctor (even if he or she is the one you overheard). Do not be afraid to ask questions! "What is the controversy about? What treatment is involved?" If you can't contact your own doctor, call the hospitalist (Rule 56). Or call any other doctor by phone—perhaps your own doctor or another doctor you know. Doctors sometimes make mistakes, and when you have warning of a possible mistake, we suggest that you not remain silent. If you are not satisfied with the answer(s) you receive, don't hesitate to change doctors. Yes, you can do so easily, particularly when you are in the hospital since there are so many doctors available. This is more feasible in a full-service or a large hospital as opposed to a small neighborhood or third-tier hospital. (See Appendix B describing various types of hospitals.)

RULE 76. WHEN TESTS ARE CONDUCTED, ALWAYS ASK YOUR DOCTOR, "WHAT DID THE TEST SHOW?"

Tests such as blood tests or X-rays are done to assist your doctor in his or her diagnosis and treatment. When you ask your doctor, "What did the latest test show?" you are increasing the odds of a successful hospital outcome for the following reasons:

- It will remind your doctor to actually read and interpret the tests. This can result in avoiding some of the *preventable* errors discussed in our introduction. One of these is the doctor neglecting or forgetting to read a test result. Remember: You are not the doctor's only patient; he or she may be required to read thirty or forty such results every day!
- It will tell you if you have a serious medical problem so you can follow through to protect yourself. Example: Let us say your doctor tells you, "There is something on your chest X-ray that we need to check; it may very well be nothing, but you do need a repeat X-ray." You are then in a position to follow through in a few days if, for some reason, you have not had the repeat X-rays. You can ask, "Doctor, when am I going to have that second X-ray that you told me about?"
- It will help your peace of mind if you are told, "The test was fine. You are in great shape."

Whatever information you obtain concerning your tests should be immediately noted on your spiral notepad or other paper that you have brought to the hospital. Be sure to record the full date (day, month, and year) of the discussion and see that this note is placed in your medical file at home after discharge. Of course, it will also help you to remember what you have been told, and you will be able to read all of these items both while you are in the hospital and weeks or months later when you are home. These notes will also be available in the future when you will be required to give doctors your medical history.

RULE 77. IF YOUR PRIVATE-DUTY NURSE IS HOSTILE, INCOMPETENT, OR OTHERWISE UNSATISFACTORY, DISCHARGE HIM OR HER PROMPTLY

Private-duty nurses are very expensive and are not usually covered by insurance. There is an ample supply of such nurses, so there is no need for you to put up with a private-duty nurse who isn't doing his or her job. But you must be careful about how and when you handle termination. Remember, the nurse may be very angry, so it is only logical to time the discharge so that the nurse leaves immediately upon discharge. Consequently, the best time to discharge an unsatisfactory private-duty nurse is at the end of a shift when you say to the nurse, "I am going to do without a nurse for the time being, and thank you for your service."

It is advisable, throughout the entire termination process, to have your advocate or one of the regular hospital nurses present, so they can see to it that the private-duty nurse leaves immediately without touching your chart, your medications, or any equipment. If you (or your advocate) have enough warning of this problem and have arranged for a replacement nurse, this person could also be asked to be present when the "firing" occurs. This will help to assure a smooth transition.

RULE 78. AVOID LOSS OR THEFT OF YOUR CELL PHONE OR SMARTPHONE

Cell phones, smartphones, and computers provide us with protection and information our parents and grandparents could never imagine: the ability to communicate 24/7 to obtain help and the ability to communicate with anyone, at any place, at any hour. So take extra care to protect this valuable lifeline. When you are in your room, keep your phone either under your pillow or otherwise out of sight—perhaps in a drawer, your hospital kit, or some other convenient location where it will be easy to reach. The bottom line is protect your phone! And don't forget to keep it charged.

RULE 79. ASK QUESTIONS IF YOU DISCOVER SURGICAL OR OTHER TREATMENT COMPLICATIONS

Most surgeries and other hospital procedures go as planned and are quite uneventful. However, sometimes there are complications, sometimes called "unexpected events," that adversely affect patients. An example would be an unintended cutting of an artery by an inexperienced surgeon. Or an erroneous overdose of therapeutic radiation due to a mathematical error by a "physicist" who works for the hospital providing the radiation. Often, not a word is said to the patient about mistakes or other occurrences. Consequently, we suggest that questions be asked after all surgeries: "Doctor, did the surgery go as planned? Were there any complications? Did anything happen that was not expected?" (Do not assume that the patient will be told if there are complications.) While there are doctors who will candidly disclose a complication and discuss it with the patient, do not count on that.

If you discover that unexpected events did occur during surgery, ask for details: "What happened? What effect will it have on me? Will more treatment or surgery be needed?" Answers to these questions will enable you to protect yourself, and you will be better able to make decisions about future actions—both medical and legal (see Rules 102–104).

RULE 80. IF YOU ARE CLEARED FOR DISCHARGE BUT FEEL TOO SICK TO LEAVE, TAKE STEPS TO APPEAL SO YOU CAN STAY IN THE HOSPITAL

Even if a patient after surgery is cleared for discharge from the hospital, he or she may feel too sick to leave, regardless of medical advice to the contrary. Remember that you must make the final decision; you do not have to accept advice that is wrong or misguided. For example, you may still be bleeding or in severe pain (which is being ignored), or you may feel faint, dizzy, or nauseous. You may know there are good reasons why you feel that you are not ready to go home. You should understand that hospitals are under intense pressure to discharge patients ASAP. Pressure may come from Medicare, from the private insurance carrier who will be footing the bill, or from the hospital "utilization" committee. But their motive is financial; it is not guided by medical considerations. They do not want you to remain in the hospital because hospital stays are very expensive—often many thousands of dollars per day! On the other hand, your interest as a patient should supersede rigid rules (primarily financial) that mandate discharge.

There are rules of law that allow you to make an appeal if you feel you are being wrongfully and prematurely discharged. This is a situation where your advocate, friend, or relative can help you to exercise this right to appeal. Of course, you may be saying to yourself (as you read this rule), "I'm not a lawyer. How do I know what to do?" Well, there are several things you can do:

1. First, discuss your concerns and symptoms with your doctor—even if he or she has signed an order for your discharge. Perhaps your doctor is not aware of the severity of your symptoms. (Or a different doctor may have ordered the discharge.)

2. You (or your advocate) can telephone the hospital administrative office and tell them, "I want to appeal the decision to discharge me."

3. If you are physically able to do so, walk to the administrative office or send your advocate and say the same.

4. Make the same request to the hospital social worker, who handles such requests.

5. Ask your doctor to help—even if he or she disagrees: "I want to appeal this discharge decision. Please help me."

It is certainly possible that your doctor is responsible for forcing your discharge. If so, despite your plea, you would probably not be able to obtain help from him or her. You might also call your family doctor and ask for help, including a second opinion from another doctor. You can also ask for a consultation by the hospitalist (Rule 56). You should not be surprised if all of the available doctors are against you, and you should be aware of another unfortunate (but not rare) medical fact: the "herd phenomenon," where if one or two senior doctors express an opinion, the others simply follow along meekly and fail to exercise their own independent judgment. It has happened time and time again. The bottom line is this: If you don't feel able to leave, do what it takes to appeal. This is also a good time for you or your advocate to call a lawyer who may be able to advise you how to exercise your rights. Above all, fight for your rights; don't give up!

RULE 81. UPON DISCHARGE, ASK FOR WRITTEN INSTRUCTIONS ABOUT MEDICATIONS OR OTHER REQUIRED ACTION

At the time of discharge from the hospital, patients are often told to take medications—perhaps postoperative antibiotics—or they may be given certain exercises to do or other instructions. Whatever the advice or instructions, they may not be easy to remember. Therefore, you should ask that you be given suggestions in writing.

If there are discharge instructions written in the chart, ask hospital personnel to make a photocopy for you of the page or pages with the instructions. If such notes are not available, ask someone in the hospital—perhaps a nurse or your doctor—to write you a note containing the instructions. Or ask that instructions be dictated into your smartphone (if you have one) as described at Rule 28. As with all other rules, be diplomatic. Simply because you are about to be discharged does not relieve you of the obligation to be courteous and friendly.

RULE 82. DO NOT SIGN ANY DOCUMENTS WHEN YOU LEAVE THE HOSPITAL

On the day of discharge, patients are often requested to sign documents that—they are usually told—are "routine." This is a simple rule—*do not sign anything*. Simply leave the hospital when you are ready to do so. You may be told that you are required "by law" or "by hospital rules" to sign. This is nonsense, and you should—courteously—say no and sign nothing. There is no law that compels you to sign any document. Nor can you be compelled to pay your bill in full or in part before you leave. There is no imprisonment for debt in the United States, and you should know this because well-meaning but misguided hospital employees may say to you, "You can't leave the hospital unless you pay your bill or sign a promise to do so." Again, this is nonsense! (It would be "imprisonment.") As indicated previously, you can leave any time you wish.

There is a good reason for this rule. Hospitals like to be paid, and if you have not already signed an agreement to pay your bill before the date of discharge, this may be the last chance the hospital has to obtain your signature on a binding obligation to pay.

If there is any bill discussion, simply say, "I will pay what I owe, but I am not going to sign anything now. If I do owe money, of course I will pay, but I will look into this after I am home."

Then simply get dressed and walk out. If you need a wheelchair, ask for one. This is a time when your advocate can help you.

5

RULES COVERING TESTS AND MEDICAL DEVICES: X-RAYS, CT SCANS, MRIS, BLOOD, URINE, AND OTHER TESTS

Rules 83–88

The following rules explain our suggestions when you are told you should have various kinds of tests, either from a mechanical instrument (X-rays, scans, MRIs, ultrasounds, EKGs, EEGs, and others) or tests involving blood, urine, or other body parts or fluids.

Today's medical equipment and testing is far more complicated than it was in years past, and these rules will help you navigate when you are told by the doctor to take these tests.

RULE 83. ASK QUESTIONS BEFORE YOU AGREE TO TESTS OR DEVICES (SEE EXCEPTIONS)

Modern medicine has developed all sorts of tests, X-rays, scans, blood examinations, and many more. Some are harmless; others—typically X-rays for a full-body scan—may expose the patient to a large amount of radiation. Of course, you should trust your doctor when he or she orders tests, but not 100 percent. We suggest that for most tests, you should ask questions before you consent:

1. Does this test (or device) pose any dangers, and if so, what are they?
2. What is the function of the test; what do you expect to find out?
3. How will it help you to make a diagnosis of my condition or decide on treatment?
4. Is there any danger to me if I don't have this test?

If the answers do not satisfy you, simply tell the doctor you would like to defer or postpone the test temporarily until you can obtain a second opinion (Rule 8).

If you are told it is dangerous to postpone the test, ask the doctor, "What is the danger?" Depending on the answer you receive, either follow your doctor's suggestion or obtain a prompt second opinion so you are able to make a decision.

Of course, you do not want to come across as a "nut," and there is no need to ask questions if the need for the test is obvious: a routine blood test (CBC) or X-rays if there is concern about a possible fracture after a bad fall or a severe auto accident. But you should definitely inquire and think carefully if multiple X-rays are ordered for a very minor injury. You should ask the doctor, "Why am I having any X-rays at all for this minor incident?"

Or let's suppose your doctor tells you that this is a "new" type of treatment or a "new" machine that he has not used before. This is another example of a warning sign indicating that you should ask questions.

RULE 84. ASK THAT ALL TESTS ORDERED BY YOUR DOCTOR BE CONDUCTED AND INTERPRETED IN THE US (SEE EXCEPTIONS)

It has become popular with many medical offices to send X-rays and blood to other countries to be analyzed. X-rays may be reviewed, for example, by a radiologist in India. However, if any of these interpretations are negligently done (pathology is missed or some other error) and if harm is caused to the patient, there is absolutely no United States legal jurisdiction, which means you would not be able to make a claim or sue for injury or damages.

In contrast, when tests or interpretations are done in the United States, our courts do have jurisdiction, and the injured patient is legally able to make a claim and sue for damages (if a lawsuit is required). While it may be true that the cost of having an interpretation done in the United States may be more than the cost of having it done in India or any other foreign country, this would be false economy. We advise our readers to make it clear that they wish to have only United States doctors and laboratories involved and not those in foreign countries. We also advise that you explain your reasoning to your doctors.

There is another good reason you should ask that tests be interpreted in the United States. In the United States, doctors must be licensed by one of our fifty states, and this assures patients that their doctor has at least a minimum amount of training in the specialty involved. For example, if it is a United States specialist in radiology (or any other specialty field), several extra years of education and training are required. But if your X-rays or blood tests are sent overseas for interpretation, it is almost impossible to determine the adequacy and competence of the training of those who are doing the interpretation. There is no way that you as a layman can verify that such foreign professionals are competent, regardless of the assurances of your physician. As with all our other rules, this rule requires no medical knowledge. If your doctor insists that any of your tests be interpreted by doctors in foreign countries, ask why. We feel there is rarely any justification for such practice, and research indicates that when doctors do utilize experts in foreign countries, it is generally done for financial and not medical reasons. It is very simple: foreign professionals work for less! The example of Josie explains both the financial and other professional implications of foreign X-ray interpretation:

Josie fell and injured her back. Her general practitioner, Dr. Sam, had X-rays taken in his office using his X-ray machine and then sent them to a radiologist in India for interpretation. The Indian radiologist charged Dr. Sam $100 for his interpretation, which was that the X-ray did not show any pathology (he found nothing wrong). Dr. Sam billed $300 to Josie's insurance carrier and pocketed the $200 difference.

However, Josie's back pain persisted, and finally she was sent by Dr. Sam for more X-rays to an X-ray specialty office in the United States in their same city. The specialist, in addition to taking more X-rays of Josie, also examined the X-rays that had been interpreted by the Indian radiologist. The United States specialist reported that Josie had a fracture that was visible in the new X-rays and also on the original X-rays that had been examined by the Indian radiologist (who simply misinterpreted the X-rays).

This error was discovered within a matter of weeks, so the only "harm," aside from a three-week delay, was the need for another X-ray (i.e., additional radiation) and the extra expense. It was not practical for Josie to even consider legal action, because the injury and damages were relatively minor. Furthermore, even if the damages were more substantial, a legal claim would not be practical for the reasons we discussed earlier in this section.

Despite the problems created by foreign interpretations, there are some important exceptions to this rule. An example of this might be a patient who suffers a severe injury at 11:30 p.m. An X-ray technician is directed by the on-duty doctor to take a complete set of X-rays, but the radiologist to interpret the X-rays does not come on duty until 7:30 a.m.—eight hours later—and this particular hospital is unable to obtain a radiologist at any earlier time. But a reading can be available within one hour from a radiologist in India (the X-rays are digital and can be sent immediately). Clearly, the patient's interests justify the foreign interpretation; prompt interpretation outweighs the risks we have discussed.

RULE 85. WHEN YOUR BLOOD IS TAKEN FOR TESTING, CHECK THAT YOUR NAME IS ON THE BODY OF THE CONTAINER

After your blood has been taken, watch to see that your blood container has your name on the *body* of the container, not the cap. Otherwise, there is the danger of mislabeling; your blood could be mixed up with the blood of another patient who will have much different medical problems than you have. Usually, the person who takes your blood—called a *phlebotomist*—will either print your name on the vial body itself or attach a preprinted label with your name on it. Then, the labels are placed on each vial. (Often three or four vials of blood are taken.) But if this is not done when the blood is taken, and if the vials are taken to another room for identification purposes, there is real danger of a mix-up. To avoid this, it is usually not necessary to do anything more than watch the labels being attached. But if you are "excused" or if the blood is about to be taken away and you have not seen your name placed on each vial, we suggest you speak up and ask questions. "I would like to be present when my name is put on each of these vials. I will feel more comfortable about it and can feel confident that there will be no mistake."

It is well known that severe health problems have been caused in the past by "later" labeling, or putting the name of the patient only on the cap, or some other error that results in mixing up one patient with another. In other words, protect yourself by being vigilant and watching what is being done. Insist on seeing to it that your name is placed on the container and not simply on the cap. The example of Dorina explains this rule:

Dorina was fifty years old. Blood was taken because there was concern that she had a serious condition involving her ovaries. Dorina didn't even understand what the problem was, but she gave her blood and left the office. Two days later, she received a call from the doctor that he had "bad news." The test indicated there was cancer and that her ovaries had to be removed promptly. Arrangements were made, Dorina went to the hospital, and her ovaries were removed.

The operation went without incident, and Dorina was relieved, since she did not expect to have more children and gave the matter no further thought.

Three months later, she received a call that requested her to make an appointment. She saw her doctor, and he said to her, "I have good news. It turns out there was a mix-up in the samples and your blood showed everything was fine. It is unfortunate that your ovaries were removed, but it was 'one of those things.'"

Dorina contacted a lawyer and did receive compensation for the negligent conduct causing the loss of her ovaries. Investigation disclosed that Dorina's name had been placed on the cap only; not the body of the container. Then her cap was switched—in error—with the cap of a different patient. This error would have been avoided if our rule had been followed.

RULE 86. WHENEVER A NEEDLE IS USED, VERIFY THAT IT IS TAKEN FROM AN UNOPENED AND STERILE PACKAGE

Routinely in the United States today in almost every medical office, a new package with a sterile needle is used for each patient, for injections and when blood is taken. Only rarely are needles reused, after sterilization by a device called an *autoclave*. Therefore, watch and you should see the technician tear open a new package to obtain a new needle. If there is any question about it and you don't see this take place, or if it has (apparently) already happened, simply ask the technician, "Is this a new sterilized needle? I didn't see the package being opened, and I've been told that I should always ask." Try to ask with a smile; no need to be hostile! If the answer is not reassuring, do not allow the needle to be used, and take your inquiry to whoever is in charge. Such action is rarely necessary, but it can happen. Remember, your health and safety are paramount, and you must act to protect yourself.

RULE 87. ALWAYS REQUEST LEAD SHIELDING FOR TESTS INVOLVING RADIATION (ALL X-RAYS AND SCANS)

This rule applies to all X-rays of any body part, including dental X-rays, CT scans, or any tests that involve radiation. We now know that X-rays can cause serious harm unless lead shielding is used to protect body parts that are not being X-rayed. Most but not all doctors and dentists use protective lead shields for their patients. These are often called lead aprons. Sometimes, if you do not ask that a lead shield be used, technicians may forget or neglect to use such protection. We suggest you be diplomatic. If you are about to be X-rayed and nothing has been done to protect your body, you should ask, "I would appreciate using lead shielding—will you please do that?" (or words to that effect). Usually, this is all that is needed. But if you were told by the doctor, technician, or nurse, "Oh, there is no need for lead shielding," or "This machine does not require such protection," we suggest you state firmly, "If there is not going to be any shielding, I don't want to be X-rayed." If this type of problem occurs to you, it is a very good reason to change doctors or dentists promptly. Radiation protection is absolutely essential, and there are no exceptions that should be allowed to this rule regardless of what you are told by any physician or radiologist.

RULE 88. IF YOU ARE TOLD TO USE A DEVICE, HAVE IT EXPLAINED TO YOU WHILE YOU ARE STILL AT THE OFFICE

You may be given a brace to use for your arm or crutches for your legs. Or you may be given a wrapping device that is not put on in the office or a "nerve stimulator" or other device. Or your doctor may request some sort of twenty-four-hour record to watch your blood pressure using some equipment. Usually, these devices are actually put on your body in the medical office. But sometimes— particularly if someone is in a hurry—you may be given directions without a hands-on demonstration. But if it is a device like a crutch, stimulator, or brace, try it out and make sure you know how to do it while you are still in the medical office. Questions can be asked in the office if necessary, and everyone saves time and avoids aggravation. Don't wait to try out these devices until you get home.

6

RULES CONCERNING MEDICATIONS AND PRESCRIPTIONS

Rules 89–96

At one time or another, all of us take medication—sometimes by prescription from our doctor and sometimes by direct purchase over the counter. There are two concepts to remember as you purchase and use your medication:

1. Buy your drugs and medications from a well-known organization in the United States. This may be your local pharmacy or it might be one of the chains like CVS, Walgreens, Rite Aid, Longs—and there are many more. Our rules explain why we suggest you try to remain with United States manufacturers. Where practical, do not buy any drugs or medications manufactured outside of the United States, although this may not always be practical. But try (Rule 89)!
2. Be cautious about purchasing any medications or prescriptions that you see advertised on television, print media, or radio (Rule 20). We suggest that you attempt to remain with drugs and medications ordered or approved by your doctor.

CHAPTER 6

RULE 89. BE CAREFUL BUYING PRESCRIPTIONS BY MAIL OR ONLINE PHARMACIES; SOME ARE GOOD, SOME ARE BAD, SOME ARE FRAUDULENT

There are many perfectly safe and legitimate mail-order pharmacies. Many seniors on Medicare using Plan D obtain all their medicine by mail from reputable national organizations. On the other hand, there are also some bogus organizations—some in the United States and some overseas—that promise to provide you with medication at a fraction of the cost you might expect. Our advice: do not buy any medication by mail or online unless you know you are dealing with a well-known national organization like CVS, Walmart, United Healthcare, Optum Rx, and others.

There are also a number of other pharmacies that operate online and also by telephone. They are aggressive and very persistent. They promise to supply all types of medications at low cost. Many of them are based in foreign countries, but they do not disclose this fact. They tell prospective buyers that they are "in the United States," and many do maintain United States addresses. Also, they almost always have names that sound American. Our advice: do not buy any drugs from these organizations, no matter how good they sound. Buy only from well-known pharmacies that are either based in the United States or that you know to be legitimate. Try to buy drugs physically manufactured in the US. But we admit this may not be possible because about half of all drugs sold in the US, by both the chains and independents, are manufactured in foreign countries, where our FDA (Food and Drug Administration) has a difficult time keeping up with inspection of drug manufacturing plants. These facilities are almost always able to claim FDA approval. But it is well known that often too many years elapse between FDA inspections.

The practical answer to this problem is to purchase only from well-known US retail pharmacies—whether chains, independents, or mail order. Sometimes, upon request, you can obtain drugs made in the US, but accept the fact that you will, very often, end up with drugs made in India (the largest generic supplier) or some other foreign country. We have carefully investigated this problem and have concluded that we must simply rely on our FDA for protection.

RULE 90. SELECT YOUR LOCAL PHARMACIES CAREFULLY; IT WILL SAVE TIME AND MONEY AND WILL PROTECT YOUR HEALTH

Even if you obtain medications by mail, most patients also patronize local pharmacies—either independents or the chains such as CVS, Walgreens, and Walmart. Here are the rules for local pharmacies:

1. Stay with well-known, reliable pharmacies. Many are not (see Rule 89).
2. Try to limit the number of pharmacies patronized. If you wish to check on an old prescription, it is much easier to do so if you have limited your purchases to one or two pharmacies.
3. Locate a convenient 24/7 pharmacy. It will be handy in an emergency on late evenings, weekends, or holidays. All the chains listed above have such pharmacies.
4. Consider a pharmacy that delivers to your home. A surprising number of pharmacies offer this service at low cost.

Note: Don't forget to obtain and keep an extra copy of each prescription for your medical file. (This will be discussed under Rule 93.)

RULE 91. IF YOU FEEL SICK OR HAVE ANOTHER PROBLEM WHEN STARTING NEW MEDICATION, STOP IMMEDIATELY AND CONTACT YOUR DOCTOR

Sometimes new medications unexpectedly cause serious reactions. Perhaps you are allergic and didn't know it. Perhaps the medication is defective. Perhaps no one knows what the problem is. But it is only common sense: if you take the medication and start to feel sick immediately, do not wait. Stop and call the doctor on an emergency basis or even go to a hospital emergency room (ER) if you can't reach a doctor. Even if the medication is wrong, dangerous, or the wrong dosage, if you stop immediately and don't simply "follow doctor's orders," you can usually avoid serious complications. Of course, along with stopping, let us again emphasize the wisdom of prompt medical attention—either from your own doctor or from any qualified emergency room or urgent care center.

Reminder: retain the medication; do not take it back or give it to anyone. Keep it in your possession because if there is any problem where a claim may have to be made on your behalf, or if a chemical analysis is needed, you do not want to lose your evidence. If your doctor wants to see the medication, certainly take it to the doctor and show it, but retain the container and its contents so you will have the evidence you need.

RULE 92. CHECK WITH YOUR DOCTOR ABOUT TAKING, CONTINUING, OR STOPPING MEDICATIONS

We offer three simple rules about how you should handle medical prescription issues.

1. Do not start, stop, or change the dose of any medication unless you first check with your doctor. (With some medications, stopping abruptly can be very dangerous.)

2. Once you begin taking any medication regularly, for more than a few weeks, at least every six months ask the prescribing doctor: "Should I continue taking this medication? For how long?"

3. As stated in Rule 20, be very wary of television ads about new and miraculous medications that promise to cure all types of problems. These ads, no matter how convincing, are simply sales pitches—pure and simple!

You may think it is strange that we have rules like the above about handling medical and prescription issues. But we remind our readers that the buck absolutely stops with them. You are the one who will suffer the consequences of taking the wrong medication, or the right medication for too long a period, or for "trying" or stopping a medication due to a persuasive sales pitch on TV. You cannot rely upon your doctors to remind you of these issues. Despite their best intentions, doctors can forget. You must remember that your doctor probably has several hundred patients and may find it difficult to keep track of who is taking what despite the most careful and conscientious charting, training of employees, and so on.

To illustrate this rule, we will look at the example of Pat, who decided to play doctor:

Pat had been on steroids for many months. She decided—on her own—to stop abruptly because she read a magazine article about the dangers of taking steroids. She did not consult her physician. She collapsed and almost died from adrenal cortical insufficiency. (This can happen if steroids are abruptly stopped.)

If the doctor wanted her to stop the medication, and if there were good medical reasons to do so, she would have been advised to taper off slowly. This would have avoided the disaster described.

RULE 93. VERIFY THAT THE MEDICATION YOU ARE TAKING WAS PRESCRIBED BY YOUR DOCTOR

There are thousands of medications that are prescribed for all types of problems: for the heart, for weight loss, for pain relief, and for many other purposes. Even physicians find it difficult to keep informed. Mistakes are frequently made, both by physicians and pharmacies. Fortunately, there are some simple steps that can be taken by you as the patient to reduce the possibility of receiving the wrong medication:

1. When you are handed a prescription by your doctor, before you have the prescription filled, be sure to retain a copy for your medical file. You can have a copy made either at the doctor's office if there is a willing helper and a copy machine, or you can make one at home if you have your own copy machine. You can even take a photo of it on your cell or smartphone providing the lens is about eighteen inches away from what you are photographing. But be sure to print a copy promptly if you do this.

2. When the doctor hands you the prescription, verify that the prescription shows your full name—and do this before you make your copy.

3. When the medication comes into your possession—whether you receive it by mail or at a pharmacy—immediately compare the medication itself with a copy of the prescription that you have retained (no. 1 above). Make sure they match, which means that the medication and the prescription slip show the same medication with the same dosage.

4. If you cannot read and/or understand the prescription when you receive it, ask that the contents of the prescription be read to you and ask for a clear explanation. Make sure you understand what you are being told.

5. If you are not handed a paper prescription but are told the prescription will be transmitted electronically from your doctor directly to the pharmacy (as is often being done), ask

that the name of the medication and the dosage be clearly written on paper and handed to you. Then, when you actually receive the medication, read the container label carefully and verify that it has your name and that it appears to be the medication that was ordered for you.

If the medication happens to be a refill, make sure the refill contains the same medication as the original prescription. There is a very good reason to keep some of your empty containers—at least until you receive a refill of the medication. This gives you the opportunity to compare the old with the new and make sure they match.

This entire process of checking medication and comparing containers can be very complicated for another reason. Different manufacturers who make precisely the same medication may produce a pill or capsule that looks different, with a different shape and different color. Also, different medications might look exactly or almost exactly alike. The following example explains what can happen if a patient does not follow this rule:

Mary was urinating with embarrassing frequency. Her family doctor wrote out a prescription for a drug called "Vesicare," which, she told Mary, would slow down her urination so she wouldn't have to constantly go to the bathroom. Mary took the prescription slip, but she did not bother to read it or make a copy of it. She simply took it to her regular pharmacy and waited for the prescription to be filled.

Unbeknownst to Mary, the pharmacist made a serious error. Although he placed Visicare (the correct medication) in the container, he made a serious mistake. He printed the instructions for a different drug with a similar name, Visicol, which is a drug designed to clean out the colon before a colonoscopy. Then, he affixed the Visicol instructions to the Vesicare container. Result: He gave Mary the correct medication (Visicare) with the wrong label (Visicol).

Since Mary did not know the name of the drug she was supposed to be taking—not having read the prescription slip—she simply followed the instructions printed on the container and took fourteen of the Visicare pills over a two-hour period. Since the correct dosage was one pill every twenty-four hours (which should have been on the label if it had been correct), this meant that Mary had taken a huge overdose—fourteen times the normal dose.

The results were disastrous. Her fluid systems shut down completely. She stopped urinating. Her eyes would not tear. There was no saliva in her mouth. Fortunately, her doctor discovered the error when Mary saw her and gave her the container. Mary's doctor took the necessary steps to restore her fluid systems, although she endured weeks of misery. Litigation followed against the pharmacy and resulted in a large settlement.

This catastrophe would have been avoided had Mary simply followed our rule. She would have retained a copy of her prescription. Or if she did not receive a paper prescription, she would have asked that the name and drug dosage be clearly written out and given to her. Then, when she received the medication, she would have compared the label on the container with the paper given her at the medical office. She would have seen that the label said "Visicol." She would have said to the pharmacist: "This looks wrong. I was supposed to receive 'Visicare,' not 'Visicol.'"

This rule explains a crucial point. When you receive medications from your pharmacy, before taking the medication you must compare the label on the container with your copy of the prescription (or a note containing the prescription information) to make sure that they match. Otherwise, you may end up with the wrong medication, like Mary in our example.

Note: There is software widely available that warns pharmacists if they have made the type of mistake that resulted in Mary's disaster. But such "protective" software must be *used* (and not overlooked or ignored). For unknown reasons, Mary received no such protection; if the software *did* warn the pharmacist, the warning was ignored. Nor did Mary properly protect herself by reading the printed consumer medication notice that every pharmacist usually hands to patients. If he did hand her reading material, she did not read it. This simply verifies one of the basic messages that we wish to convey to our readers: the buck stops with you. You must protect yourself!

RULE 94. ASK YOUR DOCTOR TO PRESCRIBE THE GENERIC UNLESS THERE ARE GOOD REASONS TO DO OTHERWISE

Brand-name medications are generally far more expensive than the generic, which, according to the law, must accomplish the same purpose and be just as effective as the brand name. Therefore, ask your doctor if a generic can be prescribed.

The catch is that brand medications are often patented, and this allows the manufacturer to retain control and ownership and charge a much larger price. Often, many years elapse before the law allows medications to be made in inexpensive generic forms. Occasionally there may be good medical reasons why you should remain with a brand medication and avoid the generic. But this is a decision that should be made by your doctor.

RULE 95. DISCARD AND REPLACE OUTDATED MEDICATIONS

When you receive medication, always check and verify that it has an expiration date, which may be one to five years. If there is no such date, ask the pharmacist to put a date on your container. You should not use medication after the expiration date, although most medical authorities state there is some leeway—perhaps two or three months.

RULE 96. DO NOT GIVE CHILDREN ADULT MEDICATION (SEE EXCEPTIONS)

Medication for an adult can be dangerous when given to children—even "standard" medication like aspirin or Tylenol, which can be habit-forming for both adults and children. (There is increasing public awareness of the dangers of pain medication.) The bottom line is to be very careful before you give adult medication to a child.

But there are exceptions. If you have an antibiotic, and there is a serious medical condition and you are out of town with your family, it is a simple matter to check with your doctor by telephone or some other doctor and find out if the medication you happen to have for yourself can also be given to children. This is an exception to this rule that would allow you, under certain unusual circumstances, to use adult medication for children.

7

FINANCIAL AND INSURANCE ISSUES

Rules 97–101

Physical survival requires you to navigate through a lifetime of medical and hospital services. If you are careful and follow our rules, you can do much to preserve your health and ability to enjoy life. But physical survival and health preservation is only half of the equation; the other, very essential piece to survival and health preservation is financial. You do not want to constantly be in debt, struggling to pay a mountain of medical and hospital bills. These are easy to create if you are ill, disabled by a serious accident, or otherwise incapacitated so you cannot earn money. The problem is that if you are sick or handicapped, those medical and hospital bills have a habit of adding up—big time.

The answer is *insurance*. Modern-day America has come to your rescue through the Affordable Care Act (ACA—sometimes called Obamacare). For the first time in our history, whether sick or well, most of us are able to buy and retain, at affordable rates, medical and hospital insurance that will pay for the diagnosis and treatment needed—whatever your medical problems. There is no longer any exclusion because of preexisting medical conditions. And you can now buy such insurance whether or not you are employed. You may also be able to obtain financial assistance from the government to help you purchase insurance. You can also change jobs or stop working altogether and still retain your insurance.

So, our first rule in this chapter concerns insurance. If you are already insured, be sure to keep your insurance unless you replace it with other insurance that will give you benefits you need—perhaps with a lower cost or better coverage. However you do it, the concept is that obtaining insurance will definitely help to assure your financial survival as well as your physical survival.

Cautionary note: Medical and hospital insurance is a complex subject. These next five rules will give you the basics, but there is much more you might learn. For a full and very informative explanation of Medicare, we urge our readers over 65 to obtain the free US government book *Medicare and You*, which is updated each year. It is available at www.medicare.gov or by calling 1-800-633-4227. Much more information can be located, without cost, online. Also, bookstores are replete with a large supply of books on the subject.

RULE 97. MAINTAIN MEDICAL, HOSPITAL, AND DRUG INSURANCE

Regardless of your age and financial status, you can now obtain affordable medical, hospital, and drug (prescription/medication) insurance. Wealthy readers may think, "I am rich. I don't need insurance at all." But you are wrong, unless you are a mega-millionaire. Why? Because a serious and long-term illness can easily cost millions or at least many thousands. It is not at all unusual for hospitals to charge $5,000 a day or more. When surgical fees and drug and other charges are added, bills of $40,000 or $50,000 for a three-day hospital stay are not at all unusual.

Medical and Hospital Coverage

As an insurance buyer, you will fall into one of the same two categories outlined in Rule 1:

A. Those Who Buy Full/Original Medicare (Medicare A for Hospitals and Medicare B for Doctors and Other Expenses)

Generally, this coverage applies to those 65 and older. But in addition to enrolling in full/original Medicare, we advise readers to purchase a Medigap policy to cover the 20 percent of Part B expenses (which can amount to many thousands) that Medicare does not cover. This can be a sizable amount of money, and those who think their basic 80 percent policy is "enough" are mistaken. After all, if a Medicare B expense (for doctor services) for $100,000 is approved for payment, Medicare pays only $80,000 and you must pay the remaining $20,000. And if your bill is larger, you will owe proportionally more.

Once you have full/original Medicare, along with the Medigap policy mentioned, every conceivable medical and hospital bill is probably covered except for a (possible) small deductible.

B. Everyone Else (Except Those with Full/Original Medicare)

It may seem strange, but this second category covers everyone else except those enrolled in full/original Medicare (category A just discussed). If you are not enrolled in full/original Medicare, you will definitely fit in one of the following sub-categories:

1. *Medicare Advantage.* This is an excellent program similar to original Medicare. But those in the Medicare Advantage program do not need to purchase a Medigap policy, which will cost $150 to $300 per month. The most significant difference between full/original Medicare and Medicare Advantage, aside from the lower cost, is the restricted ability to choose your doctor. Medicare Advantage patients may only see doctors who are in their own "network" (which is established by the insurance carrier). If a specialist is needed,

they must first consult their regular doctor (usually referred to as a "gatekeeper"), who will decide if a specialist is required. One example of a Medicare Advantage provider is Kaiser Permanente. If you are enrolled in one of their programs, you must receive your medical care from one of the doctors employed by Permanente. Generally, patients may not go outside of the Kaiser Permanente organization for care (although there are some very limited exceptions in unusual circumstances). If your Medicare Advantage plan is provided by one of the other carriers (Aetna, Travelers, Blue Cross Blue Shield, etc.), you must also utilize the doctors and hospitals that are provided by the "network" for that particular plan. Each carrier—as well as Kaiser Permanente—publishes a booklet describing their services, or they will have this information online. They also provide the names and locations of doctors who are in their networks. As mentioned above, members must select their doctor(s) from those listed in their network.

2. *Private insurance.* This classification includes many private (non-governmental) organizations, such as traditional insurance companies and all sorts of other providers, ranging from large hospitals (some of which are affiliated with medical schools), medical schools, and large private medical groups of doctors or other "hybrid" organizations. These private groups also provide complete medical and hospital care.

3. *Other government-sponsored plans—federal, state, and local.* This category covers those who cannot afford or otherwise qualify for Medicare, Medicare Advantage, or other private coverage. There are many plans that cover those who fit into this category, which handles those with lower income, those who are indigent, or those who do not fit into the other plans. The largest such group is the federal-state Medicaid program, which provides a full range of medical and hospital services for those who cannot pay or qualify for other plans we have previously discussed. These Medicaid

plans have different names in each of the states that participate in this federal/state program.

4. *United States armed forces.* This group covers the millions
   in the armed forces and their families. The United States
   armed forces—Army, Navy, Air Force, Marines, and Coast
   Guard—provide medical and hospital services all over the
   world for members of the armed forces and their families.
   Many millions of Americans receive such complete medical
   and dental care.

5. *The Veterans Administration.* The United States Veterans
   Administration has thousands of facilities throughout the
   United States and in many foreign countries. They provide
   complete care for many millions of veterans, in addition to
   certain benefits for their families.

Drug/Medication/Prescription Coverage

Regardless of your insurance plan (category A or one of the B
plans discussed), you should enroll in a plan that will pay for your
medications and prescriptions. These can be very costly if you
must pay out of pocket—particularly because many of the newer
drugs are not yet generic and there is no other way to obtain these
drugs except from the manufacturer that holds the patent (which
allows the manufacturer to keep prices very high). Almost daily,
the pharmaceutical industry is introducing these new and very
expensive drugs. They may prove to be absolutely essential to your
health because drugs today can cure or almost cure diseases that
were previously quite deadly, such as hepatitis C. Other new drugs
are of questionable value; many are simply older drugs with minor
changes in composition, but with little advantage for the patient.
Their primary purpose is to create more income for the drug manufacturers, who are able to obtain a patent for their "new" drug.
They can then set and maintain a much higher price as compared
with the older drug, which has "gone generic" and therefore
would bring in far less income. Readers should always check with

their physicians to see if they can safely remain on their "old" drug, or if they should pay the added cost of the new drug.

Before we consider how you might purchase or otherwise acquire insurance to cover drug costs, keep this fact in mind: While you are a hospital patient, all medications are covered by your hospital insurance. They are considered to be an expense like bandages, daily care, the use of operating rooms, and other expenses. But when you take medication any other time (when you are not a hospital patient), you are on your own financially, and costs can easily reach the many thousands.

There are two sources from which you may purchase medication/prescription insurance:

1. *Government—Medicare Plan D.* This coverage was created by Congress in 2003. It is a large and popular program. It is designated D to follow the other three Medicare programs—Plan A (hospital), Plan B (doctor and other expenses), and Plan C (Medicare Advantage). Patients must be enrolled in Medicare Plan A or B to be eligible for Plan D coverage, which is available to all Medicare enrollees, whether they are covered by full/original Medicare or Medicare Advantage.

2. *Private insurance.* There are many private insurance plans that provide medical and prescription coverage. Some of these plans work with unions, some work with business enterprises, and some are sold individually. We suggest that readers contact one or more of the insurance plans directly (Blue Cross Blue Shield, Aetna, etc.). All carriers have *agents* who are ready and able to explain (and sell). Readers may also contact an insurance *broker*, who has connections with many different plans. There is no cost (to readers) for such service, since insurance agents and brokers are paid by the insurance carriers.

Conclusion: Medical, Hospital, and Drug Insurance

Obtain medical, hospital, and drug insurance. If you are already insured, be sure to maintain your insurance coverage. Think carefully before you cancel, and if you do, be sure to replace it with something better. The industry has been in a state of flux in the months and years before publication of this book, but the general trend is to provide more rather than less coverage, and we expect this trend to continue.

The entire subject of insurance coverage—for medical, hospital, and drugs—is broad and complex. A detailed and more complete discussion is beyond the scope of this book. As mentioned at the beginning of this chapter, we suggest that ("original") Medicare and Medicare Advantage readers obtain the excellent and free government publication *Medicare and You*. We also suggest that anyone age 65 or older (or younger if disabled) avail themselves of free services provided by the US government at the many conveniently located Social Security offices. There are thousands all over the country that are staffed by government employees who are trained and ready to advise about all types of inquiry: Are you eligible? When to apply? How to apply? All readers pay taxes and should take advantage of these free services.

RULE 98. VERIFY IN ADVANCE THAT YOUR BILLS WILL BE PAID BY YOUR MEDICAL PLAN

The best time to protect your medical and financial future is to act well in advance and not wait until you are ill or injured, are in some accident, or experience some other medical emergency. That is not the time to discover that you have an insurance problem; they are avoided by following the preceding rule (97) and obtaining insurance coverage well in advance of medical problems, including any emergencies or other unknowns. Acting in advance, therefore, will provide the most benefit at the least cost. But even if you have followed Rule 97 and obtained the best coverage you can, you must use your insurance coverage properly. This requires that, if possible, you verify that your bills will be paid before you obligate yourself. Here is an example:

Robert, age 48, was in a serious auto collision and was rendered unconscious and awakened in the XYZ Hospital. He was told that he had a serious fracture of one leg, he would need surgery "in the next few days," and he would be in the hospital for approximately seven days. He produced his insurance information from his wallet and asked hospital personnel, "Can you make sure my Blue Cross insurance will cover my hospital and other bills?" Hospital personnel contacted Robert's carrier and assured him that the insurance would pay.

Let's review what Robert's experience tells us about avoiding unnecessary expense:

Robert had already provided himself with financial protection as we discussed in Rule 97—and this was before he had any medical problem (no one knows if and when an emergency such as an accident will occur).

If there was an insurance problem when the hospital called Blue Cross, Robert and the hospital would know this before his surgery (which would be occurring within a matter of days). This indicates that Robert had time, if required, to transfer to another hospital that would accept his insurance. If Robert had not verified his coverage, and if that hospital turned out not to be "in network," Robert could have been on the hook for a $50,000-plus hospital bill—clearly a terrible financial blow.

There is really nothing more Robert could have or should have done. He had wisely planned in advance by having insurance coverage.

We realize that Robert in our example may not be the typical patient; he showed an unusual ability to think clearly even though he had been hospitalized after severe trauma. But even the more average patient should be able to take the very simple and logical step of making sure his or her medical expenses will not be paid "out-of-pocket."

Here is another example that explains how patients can avoid nasty financial surprises:

Doris, age 65, consulted a cosmetic surgeon about having a facelift; she wanted to eliminate facial wrinkles that "make me look old." She consulted Dr. Joel, who told her that his fee was $5,000, but he said, "I think your insurance will pay for this."

He had Doris sign many documents that she did not bother to read. (If she had read the documents, she would have seen that she had promised to personally pay if her insurance did not do so.) Her surgery was set at a local hospital for the following week.

Before leaving the office, Doris said, "Before I go to the hospital for my facelift surgery, would you please check to make sure that my insurance will pay all the bills—yours and the hospital's?" The doctor agreed.

Two days later, Dr. Joel's office called Doris and told her she would have to pay cash because her insurance company said this was cosmetic surgery, and that neither the doctor's fee nor the hospital bill was covered by her policy. Doris canceled the surgery and decided to live with her wrinkles.

By following this rule, Doris saved many thousands of dollars. Her desire to have a facelift was purely elective and was simply out of the question financially. Of course, if Doris had unlimited funds (multimillionaire, etc.), she could have paid the $5,000 for the surgery, plus the hospital bill, but very few patients are so fortunate.

RULE 99. REDUCE OUT-OF-POCKET EXPENSES BY BARGAINING, COORDINATING, AND SHOPPING

In this third millennium, almost all of us in the United States (citizens and legal residents) can buy insurance through the federal Affordable Care Act (ACA). And although there will undoubtedly be future changes, it appears that we no longer need be concerned about insurance carriers excluding those with preexisting medical problems.

But financial problems remain, and they will not go away. Almost all insurance plans have *deductibles*, and these tend to become larger, not smaller, as insurance carriers watch their bottom line. This means that you the patient must pay $300 to $3,000 or more in each calendar year before your insurance kicks in. X-rays, CT scans, MRIs, and other services cost hundreds or thousands of dollars; but there are three methods to use to help you save money—and remember this is your money that must be paid out of your pocket. We call these methods *bargain*, *coordinate*, and *shop*.

Bargain

Don knew that his insurance had an annual deductible of $2,000. This means that Don must personally pay that amount before his insurance kicks in. He was told that he needed to have an MRI and was directed to a nearby facility. Before he contacted the office recommended by his doctor, he made calls to two other facilities in the city that performed MRIs. He had heard from a friend that many of these tests had no fixed price (and that Medicare, Medicaid, and insurance companies always paid less). Don called the first facility and was told that the cost would be $3,000. The second place told him the cost would be $2,500. Then Don called the facility chosen by his doctor, and when he asked the price, he was told that the MRI would cost $2,000. Don told the intake person, "Look, I am paying this out of my own pocket and my doctor referred me. Can I make a deal to pay so much a month?" He was told that this laboratory would not make that type of arrangement. Don persisted and spoke to the manager, who told him that this office did not accept installment payments, but they would reduce the cost to $1,200 if Don would pay the entire amount up front. When Don explained he did not have that much cash available, they suggested that he put the bill on his credit card. Don reluctantly agreed.

Don's example explains some important points: First, it is possible to bargain and save considerable sums of money. Second, since Don decided to put the bill on his credit card, there will be substantial credit card interest on the unpaid amount (unless he pays his credit card bill in full each month). Such interest can be very expensive—10 percent to 20 percent per annum or even more. But, the reduction of the bill—down to $1,200—made the deal worthwhile.

Those who bargain should consider one other fact. You need to obtain your doctor's okay for any organization where you are able to bargain and obtain a favorable price. If your doctor tells you, "Look, I know you can obtain a test (like an MRI) from XYZ Labs for much less than the lab I sent you to, but I don't trust this lab." Fortunately, Don did not have this problem because he was able to make a deal with the lab recommended by his doctor.

Coordinate

Joe, age 49, bought insurance available through ACA, for which he paid $146 per month. His deductible was $2,000 per calendar year. In November, almost eleven months after he bought the insurance policy, he fell in his bathroom and fractured his right hip, which required hospitalization and surgery. The doctor told Joe that the surgery was successful and he would be able to walk without problems. Joe was relieved. But his bills were in the many thousands, and he was required to pay his $2,000 deductible.

In early December, while Joe was recuperating at home, his doctor told him, "I want you to get a special X-ray series including a lung scan. There is something I want to check on your right lung, but there is no rush." Joe was tired of medical problems and was looking forward to attending a Christmas party for his twenty-two-year-old son who was about to be married. He made an appointment in early January; the X-rays would be expensive and would cost $4,000. He told a friend, who said, "Don't wait until next year for those tests. Have them done before December 31 of this year, and they won't cost you anything. Your insurance company will have to pay the entire bill."

The friend was right. Deductibles are computed by the calendar year. Therefore, Joe would save $4,000, their total cost, if he completed the tests by December 31, since he had already met his deductible for that year.

Joe's example illustrates how bunching expenses together in one year can save a large sum of money simply by coordinating your deductibles.

Shop

Like any other product or service, it usually pays to shop and compare prices, and health, medical, and drug coverage is no exception. But when you shop and compare prices, make sure that you are comparing like services. This is much easier to do under the ACA as well as the various Medigap insurance plans that pay the 20 percent of Medicare expenses not paid by Medicare Plan B (doctor and other services—see Rule 97). Under federal law, each of the Medigap plans—A, B, C, D—must offer identical benefits, but their premium costs may differ and depend upon what the insurance carriers wish to charge. So it pays to shop!

Likewise, under the ACA, insurance companies offer "Platinum," "Gold," "Silver," and "Bronze" plans. Like the Medigap plans, the benefits must be the same, even though many different companies sell them, but the premiums can be set at any amount the carriers wish. So, again, it will pay to shop and compare prices.

RULE 100. WHETHER YOU HAVE INSURANCE OR NOT, LEARN TO FINANCIALLY NAVIGATE OUT-OF-POCKET, OUT-OF-NETWORK, AND CONCIERGE MEDICAL PLANS

Increasingly, doctors in this third millennium are searching for methods to maintain or increase their incomes, and all readers should be aware of this phenomenon. Why? Because MDs throughout the United States are being financially squeezed by insurance carriers, Medicare, Medicaid, and all other entities that pay for medical services. In addition, there is constant pressure on doctors by federal and state entities, legislatures, and governors to improve the quality of medical care and reduce medical and hospital costs. To further complicate the national medical picture, remember that there are many millions of new patients who are now entitled to medical insurance under the federal Affordable Care Act (ACA), often referred to as Obamacare. Also, changes to the ACA may be made by the political party in power. As this book goes to press, the Trump administration is attempting radical changes; the Democrats are resisting.

These factors now exert pressure on doctors to see more patients and to charge less, as well as pressure on the insurance industry to cover more patients without increases in premiums.

Following are responses by doctors and the insurance industry to such pressures, as well as an explanation of the choices that patients can consider that are outside of traditional insurance plans:

Concierge Medical Care, Also Known as "Boutique," "Retainer," or "Personalized" Medical Care (Names May Differ)

In concierge plans, each patient pays a monthly or annual amount of money over and above the amount paid for their medical insurance, including Medicare. In return for this extra amount of money (paid directly to the doctor), patients are told that they will receive extra services not covered by their insurance. These extra services may include 24/7 access to the doctor through his or her private cell phone, at any hour of the day or night, including evenings, weekends, and holidays. Also, concierge patients may be told they will not have to endure long waits to see the doctor; they will be seen promptly. In addition, other extra services may be offered, such as dietary advice. The cost of such concierge service ranges from $50 to $200 per month. It is certainly a service to be considered for those who wish to afford the described services, although our investigation discloses that it is questionable whether such "extras" result in improved medical care.

Out-of-Pocket Plans—Not Covered by Insurance

Increasingly, there are physicians who do not accept any insurance (including Medicare) for payment of their bills. These physicians explain that their patients must pay directly; they neither request nor receive any funds from insurance. Some of these private medical plan doctors will help their patients with paperwork to attempt partial reimbursement from their insurance carrier (or Medicare). Other such physicians inform their patients that they will not be involved—at all—in helping with their patients' reimbursement efforts, except for providing a bill for their services. If patients do have insurance of some type, patients may submit these bills to their plan, and there may be some type of reimbursement, although it depends upon the plan involved (private insurance, Medicare, etc.).

The cost of such private medical care varies. Some physicians charge for each visit; others give a blanket cost of $100 to $150 a month or more. There does not seem to be any particular going rate. Nor do these plans offer total care. If the patient needs to see a specialist such as a urologist or a cardiologist, requires hospitalization and surgery, or needs any other service outside the expertise of the doctor, the patient must see such a doctor on his or her own and pay the cost, or submit it to their insurance carrier (assuming they have insurance).

Because of the limitations discussed, even our wealthiest readers should definitely maintain their own insurance coverage, because surgical and hospital expenses can easily run into the millions. Clearly, this type of plan is for readers with substantial assets that will permit this considerably larger expense.

Out-of-Network Options

No matter which insurance plan you have—whether from Medicare, Medicare Advantage, private insurance, Veterans Administration, or one of the other government plans covering servicemen—at times you may wish to go outside of your plan network or the permitted services for personal reasons. You may wish to see a particular specialist to obtain a second opinion (which was refused by your insurance carrier or other provider). Or you may wish to acquire a special crutch or wheelchair that your plan will not supply. Remember that even if you are enrolled in "original" Medicare, there are services and devices that will not be covered despite the fact that original Medicare does provide very broad coverage. An example would be an experimental treatment or drug still in FDA trials and not yet approved. If there is some question about whether a service or device will be covered, readers are advised to find out, in advance, if they must pay "out of pocket" (personally).

Sometimes your insurance plan will pay a portion of the bill for an out-of-network doctor. This is most applicable to private plans who have their own networks. Some insurance plans will pay 50 percent of the cost of an out-of-network doctor; others may pay different amounts. Members of the plan can determine what benefits are provided by either going online, reading printed publications provided by their plan, or inquiring by telephone. Almost every plan allows telephone inquiry—usually by an "800" number—although we concede that you must persevere to reach a live person.

RULE 101. BE CAUTIOUS BEFORE PUTTING OTHER MEDICAL OR LABORATORY BILLS ON YOUR CREDIT CARD

Rules 55 and 62 dealt with the hospital paperwork that a patient must review and sign before hospital entry. These rules warn patients about the dangers of signing credit card authorizations that may be buried in voluminous forms that the patient is told to sign before entry into the hospital. But there are many other medical expenses (apart from hospital bills) that can cost thousands of dollars—expenses that are incurred by patients at private laboratories that may be located inside or outside the hospital premises. Examples would be a laboratory analyzing blood (or other fluids) or an X-ray laboratory, both of which perform services for hospital inpatients and outpatients. Many of these facilities are independent legal entities that perform laboratory and other work for hospitals, as well as for those who are sent by physicians. These patients—who do not stay overnight—are simply sent to these laboratories or other facilities by their doctors with a prescription for tests such as X-rays, MRIs, or CT scans. Assuming that no emergency is involved, be very careful about signing credit card authorizations for such services. It is far better for your pocketbook to follow Rules 99 and 100 (shopping, bargaining, coordinating, etc.), which may help you to avoid thousands of dollars in unnecessary expense. Of course, once you have made your deal for the service and know what you have agreed to pay, it is perfectly logical to put the bill on your credit card, knowing that you must pay in full and will not (in all probability) be able to pay less in dealing with your credit card organization. (See Rules 55 and 62.)

8

MEDICOLEGAL ISSUES
Rules 102–104

This is our shortest chapter and contains only three rules. But these rules influence your legal as well as your financial survival. They are closely linked to the other doctor and hospital rules—particularly to the financial and insurance issues discussed in chapter 7.

A patient who is seriously injured because of a preventable medical error may incur many thousands of dollars of medical and hospital expenses. In addition, there may be very substantial lost income in the hundreds of thousands of dollars or more. If the preventable errors result in death, as discussed in the introduction, the families of victims will need evidence to prove their claims. So whether patients are injured by preventable errors and survive or whether death results, the following three rules are designed to protect their rights:

RULE 102. IF INJURY OR ILLNESS MAY HAVE BEEN CAUSED BY MEDICAL OR HOSPITAL ERRORS, OR OTHER CAUSES, TAKE STEPS TO PROTECT YOUR LEGAL RIGHTS

Unfortunate events do occur, both in doctors' offices and in hospitals. A patient can fall out of a hospital bed when protective side rails are not kept up by the nursing staff. A patient may pass out in a doctor's office after a penicillin injection. A hospital patient can fall to the floor and fracture his or her hip when the patient slips from the grasp of a nurse's aide. You—the patient—are not a lawyer. You can't be expected to know if the cause of the incident was a simple mistake without fault by a doctor or someone else. You have no way of knowing if there is legal liability by anyone. But if there is any suspicion whatsoever by you or anyone helping you, like your 24/7 advocate, that the doctor or one of his or her employees or one of the hospital personnel was at fault, or that some defective piece of equipment caused the injury, we suggest that you take simple steps to protect your legal rights:

1. If you are able to do so, immediately make a detailed, dated written note. Write it in your own handwriting—or computer or smartphone if you happen to have one with you—and describe what occurred. At your earliest convenience, see that it is printed and placed in your personal medical file. (See Rule 25.)

2. If the incident occurs in a hospital, aside from making your own note about what happened, ask a nurse or doctor to make a note in the hospital chart and to "please describe what has occurred." The doctor or hospital employee may be reluctant to make such a note, for fear of criticism by hospital authorities. But if you insist, usually some note will be made—if not on your own chart then in some other hospital record where at least there will be some notification that something occurred. This will make it more difficult for hospital personnel to deny that the incident did occur. If

you have an advocate with you in the hospital (Rule 42), ask this person to help you ask someone in the hospital to make a note of your injury, illness, or other problem.

3. If the incident or problem occurs at a doctor's office, similar action should be taken: ask your doctor or anyone else in the medical office to record the incident in your chart. Of course, you should also make your own note as indicated in number 1 above and put the information in your medical file when you return home.

4. If the incident involves evidence that is visible, such as a broken or defective chair, bed, side rail, or some other device, try to take several different photos from different angles. Every cell phone has a camera that will adequately handle this problem.

5. Obtain and record the name, telephone number, and email address of any possible witness. For example, there may be a cooperative hospital nurse, nurse's aide, or tech. There may be a patient in a nearby bed. Or someone—even a stranger—may have happened to be in the room when the incident occurred. Whoever it is, make a definite attempt to find and record the identity, telephone number, address (if possible), and email address for future reference. Remember, you will have a pen and pad in your hospital kit (Rule 51).

6. If you notice that there is some written document that is involved in your care—perhaps a note that was made in your hospital chart, a notation on a slip of paper, or any other note—also take steps to photograph this. Most cell phones will even take a readable photo of a document if the phone is positioned about eighteen inches from the document involved. This evidence can be very important later if there is a claim and possible litigation is involved.

RULE 103. IF ILLNESS OR INJURY OCCURS, AS DISCUSSED IN RULE 102, DECLINE REQUESTS FOR "INTERVIEWS" OR "STATEMENTS," AND AVOID OTHER COMMUNICATIONS THAT MAY COMPROMISE YOUR LEGAL RIGHTS

Unexpected events like injuries, illnesses, or falls may occur while you are a patient, whether in the hospital or at your doctor's office. Such negative events may also involve a pharmacy (or drug manufacturer) who supplied the wrong medication or a nurse who administered the wrong medicine. Often, these events will cause the involvement of insurance carriers and their claims personnel or members of the "risk management" staff at the hospital. It is their job to investigate and gather evidence, since they are aware that a claim might be made by the patient. The primary purpose of such personnel, who are usually well-trained and competent, is to protect the doctors, hospitals, or drug companies against claims by patients. Therefore, it is wise to decline making any kind of statement or interviewing with an investigator or risk management personnel. Remember that these investigations are not carried out to help the patient, but are carried out primarily to protect the legal interests of the hospital, doctor, or insurance carrier involved.

When these investigators or other personnel present themselves to the patient, they usually identify themselves as one of the following:

- An "investigator"
- A concerned "hospital helper" or someone affiliated with the hospital who is looking into the matter
- An employee of the hospital "risk management office"
- An insurance carrier "representative" or "adjuster"
- A hospital "volunteer" who is "concerned" and wants to "help"

These persons will ask questions and will often carry a recording device, which may be concealed. They may make written notes and then explain they have prepared a statement for your signature. Remember that they are trying to collect the same information we've already suggested: the names of witnesses, those people in other beds, and any other information you have. But no matter how major or minor the injury, how it occurred or what you are asked, our rule is the same. Give no information. Tell them you do not wish to be "interviewed" and you do not wish to discuss the incident. Be very courteous and explain that you will furnish information through your attorney or other representative at a future date. Ask for their card so that you can have someone contact them as soon as possible. Remember: You are not legally required to speak to anyone. So, be pleasant but firm in your refusal. The example of Ethel explains this rule:

Ethel, age 78, was in the hospital for a few days to stabilize her blood pressure, which had gone dangerously high. Her cardiologist told her, "Don't worry, we'll get your medication straightened out. It will take a few days, but then you'll be fine." She was under sedation and sleeping satisfactorily. Her doctor had ordered that the side rails on her bed should be kept up at all times except when she was helped to the bathroom. Ethel went to sleep at about 10:30 p.m., and the next thing she was aware of was when she woke up on the floor next to her bed. A nurse suddenly appeared; Ethel was not sure who had called her.

The nurse exclaimed, "You must have fallen out of bed—your side rails were down." Ethel was taken to X-ray and diagnosed with a fractured hip. She was examined by an orthopedic specialist, treated, and put back in bed. The side rails were raised to prevent any further falls.

Later, a young man appeared in Ethel's room. He said, "My name is Evan, and I am with risk management in the hospital. I'd like to take a statement from you with this recorder about what happened."

Ethel's son was a veteran personal-injury attorney and had briefed Ethel about what to do if anything went wrong in the hospital. Ethel told Evan, "Well, thank you for coming, but I am not going to give any statement, recorded or otherwise. Just give me your card, and I'll have my attorney call you." She smiled at Evan and said, "I'm sure you and my attorneys can work this out."

She did not tell Evan about the statement of the nurse regarding the side rails. Nor did she say she had already recorded in her own notes the name of the nurse who made the statement about the side rails and that she had also obtained the name, address, telephone, and email of the other occupant of her two-person room. In short, Ethel followed this rule.

RULE 104. EMPLOY AN ATTORNEY ASAP IF YOU BELIEVE YOU ARE A VICTIM OF MEDICAL OR HOSPITAL ERROR OR OTHER CAUSES DISCUSSED IN RULE 102

It is never easy for a patient to consider hiring a lawyer to make a claim for injury or illness due to a medical mistake or error. But if you believe you are the victim of such conduct, you should definitely consider employing a lawyer who is experienced in representing clients with such problems. Lawyers are usually employed on a "contingency basis," which means that there is no charge for their services unless the lawyer is able to obtain a financial recovery for the patient. But whether the event occurs in or out of the hospital or in a doctor's office or elsewhere, it is wise to consider prompt employment of a lawyer if the injury is significant.

If the injury occurs while you are a hospital inpatient, do not wait until discharge. It is advisable to employ an attorney while you are still hospitalized, because at that time—while you are still a patient in your hospital room—witnesses, records, and visual evidence will be much more available. For example, photographs can be taken of you, the patient, in the hospital bed (along with bandages and other implements). This can depict the setting where the injury occurred. Witnesses may also be available, such as friendly nurses or aides or other persons in the room, perhaps other patients or visitors. Experienced attorneys and their investigators will be able to ask questions and talk to possible witnesses.

But speed is essential. A witness/patient in a bed nearby might be discharged or moved within hours or the next day.

We realize it is not easy to obtain competent legal help so quickly, particularly when you may be weakened physically as well as not being in full possession of your mental faculties (due to medication or otherwise). This is the time that an advocate (Rule 42), family, or friends can be helpful; they can assist in prompt employment of legal help.

APPENDIX A

Healthcare Providers (HCPs)

Although readers usually think of MDs (medical doctors) as healthcare providers, many other persons also provide or participate in the provision of healthcare. Most of them are professionals licensed by one of our fifty states. Such licensing does provide patients with significant protection, since all states require some degree of education and training. But despite licensing requirements, the lay patient has almost no practical ability to answer a simple question: Is this healthcare provider (HCP) competent to provide the care I require? Our book explains how you, the lay patient without medical training, can best make this decision. We also explain how to deal with each of these healthcare providers.

Following is a listing of the various providers that you are likely to encounter. For those who desire more information, we suggest that computer-savvy readers use the many available search engines described in Rules 17 and 19. A surprisingly complete and accurate source of information is Wikipedia. It is clear and easy to understand. Here are the HCPs:

Doctors of Medicine (MDs)

Generally, these are the most reliable healthcare providers. They receive many years of education and training as compared to the other HCPs that we will list. We do not mean to disparage non-MDs. We simply recognize that the MD receives many years of medical education and training. This means that, as a general rule, they can be relied upon for diagnosis and treatment.

Doctors of Podiatric Medicine (DPMs)

These providers diagnose and treat disorders of the foot and ankle and do not generally deal with any other bodily structures. They receive specific, but limited, medical training focused on their narrow area of expertise.

Doctors of Dentistry (DDSs)

Dentists diagnose and treat problems involving teeth and gums.

Chiropractors (Doctors of Chiropractic)

These providers believe that disease is caused by abnormal function of the nerve system and that restoration can be achieved by manipulation of bodily parts, particularly the spinal column. As compared with MDs, readers should realize that these providers possess far less medical knowledge and training.

Physician Assistants (PAs) and Nurse Practitioners (NPs)

The training and experience of those in this group varies widely, depending on the differing laws in our fifty states. Some of these HCPs are well trained; others are not. If you are receiving care from a PA or NP, your best protection is to verify that their diagnosis and treatment is reviewed or approved by an MD.

Registered Nurses (RNs) and Licensed Vocational Nurses (LVNs)

Their usual contact with patients occurs at hospitals. But these HCPs are often also employed in medical offices outside of hospitals. At both locations, they assist physicians in day-to-day medical practice. RNs receive more education and training as compared to LVNs, but both of these professionals provide important services in caring for patients. However, like all other non-MD HCPs, they require supervision by MDs.

Physical Therapists, Sometimes Called Physio-Therapists (PTs)

These providers remedy bodily impairment and disease using a variety of physical, mechanical, and electrical methods: massage, heat packs, mechanical and electrical devices, and physical exercise.

Medical Assistants, Techs, Nurses' Aides, Medical Orderlies, and Other Medical and Hospital Employees

Some of these are licensed; some are not. It is difficult for the lay patient to evaluate their ability. If there is a question, verify their actions are supervised or approved by an MD.

APPENDIX B

Hospitals and Other Facilities That Provide Similar Services: Emergency Rooms (ERs), Ambulatory Surgical Centers, Urgent Care, and Walk-in Clinics

The odds are that sometime in your life, you or a family member will be a patient in a hospital, emergency room, urgent care clinic, or some other medical facility apart from the offices of your regular doctor. If there is no emergency, you will have time to make inquiries and participate in selecting the facility. Or an emergency may occur (911, etc.), and you will have very little input about where you (or a family member) are taken (see Rule 18).

If you do have a say in selection, it is important that you understand what services these seven facilities do (and do not) provide. For example, if you have decided upon elective (or any other nonemergency) surgery, you could ask your physician to refer you to a surgeon who operates at a full-service hospital (Rule 41). If your surgeon insists on performing your surgery at a second- or third-tier hospital, you have the option of employing a different surgeon (Rule 44).

If you need emergency care and have no control where you are taken, you will at least have an understanding of what services are available and what limitations you face.

Following is a brief description of the seven types of hospitals and similar facilities that are available to you (and your loved ones). We do concede that your power to choose is limited.

1. FULL-SERVICE HOSPITALS (FIRST-TIER, TERTIARY, OR QUATERNARY-CARE HOSPITALS)

These hospitals offer a full range of services. Specialists are available on short notice in every field: surgery, orthopedics, neurosurgery, nephrology, cardiology, infectious diseases, and others. They have well-trained, fully staffed, and well-equipped emergency departments (ERs) and intensive care units (ICUs) with prompt access to the hospital specialists.

The services of your regular attending doctor are also supplemented—24/7—by residents, interns, and their supervising physicians, most of whom are usually affiliated with major university medical schools. In addition, many of these hospitals now provide services by a physician called a "hospitalist." This is an experienced physician who is on staff 24/7 and can pinch hit if your attending doctor is not available, and if the patient requires medical services beyond the expertise of residents and interns. The equipment of these hospitals is usually complete and up to date. If the patient wishes, most of these hospitals allow the patient to bring an advocate to remain in the hospital room (Rule 42). These hospitals are preferred for all patients and all medical problems.

2. SECOND-TIER (REGIONAL) HOSPITALS

Although many of these hospitals are large and well equipped, their supply of specialists is limited as compared with full-service hospitals. Many of these hospitals do have ERs and ICUs, but the training and expertise of their personnel may be inferior to full-service hospitals. Patients can experience long and dangerous delays at such facilities while attempts are made to locate qualified specialists. Few of such hospitals are affiliated with medical teaching institutions, so there are usually no residency or intern programs. Some of these hospitals allow advocates (Rule 42) to remain with patients; others do not. There is a very wide variation in the quality of hospital services offered, but you—as a potential patient—would have difficulty in determining which offer adequate services and which do not. If there is a choice, full-service hospitals are definitely superior and preferred over these second-tier hospitals.

3. THIRD-TIER (LOCAL NEIGHBORHOOD) HOSPITALS

These are far less desirable as compared with either the full-service or second-tier hospitals described above. Some of these hospitals have ERs and ICUs, but if there are complications, specialists are even less available. There are generally no resident or intern staffs since these are not teaching hospitals. Most will not allow advocates to remain with patients. Some of these third-tier hospitals are utilized because they are close to the doctor's office. Physicians find them convenient because they are able to move back and forth between the hospital and their offices with little lost time. Like the second-tier hospitals, there is wide variation in the quality of care offered. As a general rule, these hospitals should definitely be avoided if the patient has a choice.

4. AMBULATORY SURGICAL CENTERS

These are specialty facilities focused on particular procedures—such as colonoscopies, endoscopic examination of the gastrointestinal tract, cystoscope examinations of the urinary tract, and others. They are often well equipped and staffed by very competent and experienced physicians, but their expertise is focused only on the special services they provide. Such limitation of expertise may be dangerous if serious complications arise with a patient if emergency procedures, such as complex surgery for an unexpected problem, are needed. An example would be a torn bowel requiring immediate major surgery to prevent infection. These facilities are not equipped and staffed to handle such a problem as compared to full-service hospitals. They suffer from the same lack of immediate availability of specialists as the second- and third-tier facilities previously discussed. However, for the limited services they offer, they are certainly acceptable as long as no complications arise.

5. STAND-ALONE EMERGENCY ROOMS

These ERs are not connected with any hospital. Previously, some of them may have been hospitals that later elected to stop providing services to inpatients. Some may be very well staffed with trained personnel certified in emergency medicine; others may have doctors with far less training. Like the second- and third-tier hospitals previously discussed, such ERs have no convenient access to specialists who may be required in an emergency, and there is no practical way that a non-doctor can judge their safety or competence. Valuable time can be lost by patients who require transfer to a full-service hospital. It is far preferable, if emergency services are needed for a patient, to obtain ER services in an emergency room located in a full-service hospital.

6. URGENT CARE AND WALK-IN CLINICS

These are "hybrid" offices that provide both emergency and general medical services—usually to those who do not have established doctor-patient relationships or those who have been in an accident or other emergency situations where there is no other medical help immediately available. These facilities are strictly interim locations, and patients usually will require transfer from such facilities to inpatient hospitals if there is any serious medical problem. Some of the staff personnel may be very competent and others less so. But, again, the patient will have no way of knowing, and it is impractical to investigate such matters, particularly if patients are in an emergency situation where they need medical care and the only facilities available are one of these "walk-in" facilities. These urgent care/walk-in clinics, although fulfilling a definite function, are the least desirable of all the facilities discussed if hospital services are needed.

7. HEALTHCARE PROVIDER SERVICES PROVIDED BY PHARMACIES AND OTHER RETAIL ESTABLISHMENTS

A surprisingly large number of medical services are now available and are performed, on the premises, for retail customers of pharmacies, department stores, grocery chains, and others. Establishments that provide these services include CVS, Rite Aid, Walgreens, Walmart, some of the large grocery chains, and others. Various types of services are provided to treat minor illnesses, to provide vaccinations (for flu, pneumonia, and shingles), to treat skin problems, to provide cholesterol and diabetes screening, and many others.

Readers should be aware of one significant limitation with the health services provided by such establishments. There are no physicians (MDs) involved, so all services are performed without medical supervision. If a physician is required, the nurse practitioner or physician's assistant (NP or PA) will refer the patient to an MD at some other location—hopefully nearby and without delay. Often, the referring establishment has a list of physicians to whom they refer, depending on the medical problem. But most medical problems are handled by the NP or PA without referral, as illustrated by the example of Leslie:

Leslie had a painful sore throat. It hurt her to swallow. It was a Saturday afternoon, and she knew there would be a problem reaching her regular doctor. She also knew, from prior experience, that the nearby hospital emergency department would be jammed wall-to-wall. So she went to her local CVS pharmacy and checked in with their "minute clinic." She was soon seen by the nurse practitioner (NP). Using a swab, the NP took a specimen from Leslie's throat. She left Leslie for a few minutes. She returned from their on-premises lab and said to Leslie, "It's a good thing you came in. You have a strep infection." She gave Leslie a prescription for an appropriate antibiotic, which Leslie had filled at the pharmacy on the premises. She started the antibiotic immediately.

Besides obtaining prompt care, Leslie gained one other advantage by going to the retail pharmacy clinic at CVS. She was not required to wait for twenty-four to forty-eight hours for the analysis by the laboratory to find out that she had a strep throat. The pharmacy was able to promptly obtain the necessary laboratory information and diagnose and treat this serious problem without delay.

APPENDIX C

Corrected Surgical Consent Form

1. I, *(name of patient)*, understand, request, and consent to the performance of the following operation(s) or special procedure by doctor(s) *(name of doctors ~~or his/her designee and those under his/her immediate responsibility and supervision~~)*: *(description of surgical/procedure)*

2. Further, I hereby authorize and consent to the provision of such additional services for me as they may deem reasonable and necessary, including, but not limited to the administration and maintenance of anesthesia and the performance of services involving pathology, radiology, and photography.

3. My doctor(s) have explained that the operation(s) or procedure(s) listed above may be beneficial in the diagnosis or treatment of my condition.

4. The hospital pathologist is hereby authorized to use his/her discretion in the disposition of any member, organ, or other tissue removed from my person during the above-named procedure(s).

5. I further understand that the Medical Center maintains personnel and facilities to assist my surgeon(s) and physician(s) in their performance of various surgical operations and other special

procedures. I understand that these operations and procedures may all involve risks of unsuccessful results, complications, injury, or even death from both known and unforeseen causes and no warranty or guarantee is made as to result or cure. I know that I have the right to be informed of such risks, as well as the nature and purpose of the operation or procedure and the available alternative methods of treatment and this form is not a substitute for such explanations, which are provided by the above-named physicians. Except in cases of emergency or exceptional circumstances, operations or procedures will not be performed until I have had the opportunity to receive such explanation.

6. I understand that I have the right to consent to or refuse any proposed operation or procedure any time prior to its performance. My signature below constitutes my acknowledgment (1) that I have read and agreed to the foregoing; (2) that the proposed operation(s) or procedure(s) have been satisfactorily explained to me and that I have all the information that I desire; and (3) that I hereby give my authorization and consent.

(Signature of Patient or Representative)
(Date/Time)
(Relationship to Patient)
(Witness/Date/Time)

BIBLIOGRAPHY AND
SUGGESTED READING

Bailey, Elizabeth. *The Patient's Checklist: 10 Simple Hospital Checklists to Keep You Safe, Sane & Organized.* New York: Sterling, 2012.

Brawley, Otis Webb, with Paul Goldberg. *How We Do Harm: A Doctor Breaks Ranks about Being Sick in America.* New York: St. Martin's Press, 2012.

Cohen, Elizabeth. *The Empowered Patient: How to Get the Right Diagnosis, Buy the Cheapest Drugs, Beat Your Insurance Company, and Get the Best Medical Care Every Time.* New York: Ballantine Books, 2010.

Ehrenclou, Martine. *The Take-Charge Patient: How You Can Get the Best Medical Care.* Santa Monica: Lemon Grove Press, 2019.

James, John T. "A New Evidence-Based Estimate of Patient Harms Associated with Hospital Care." *Journal of Patient Safety* (2013).

Makary, Marty. *Unaccountable: What Hospitals Won't Tell You and How Transparency Can Revolutionize Health Care.* London: Bloomsbury Press, 2012.

Michelson, Leslie D. *The Patient's Playbook: Find the "No Mistake Zone."* New York: Knopf, 2015.

Pronovost, Peter, and Eric Vohr. *Safe Patients, Smart Hospitals.* New York: Penguin Group Hudson Street Press, 2010.

Wen, Leana, and Joshua Kosowsky. *When Doctors Don't Listen: How to Avoid Misdiagnoses and Unnecessary Tests.* New York: St. Martin's Press, 2014.

INDEX

perform surgery (rule 67), 91–92;
take steps to appeal if not ready for
discharge (rule 80), 102–103; tell
surgeon about dentures, implants,
or stents (rule 69), 93; verify body
warning signs are placed and visible
(rule 66), 91; verify medication
(rule 72), 95–96

rules when elective or non-emergency
surgery and hospitalization are first
considered, 41–42; arrange to have
advocate/friend in hospital room
(rule 42), 55–58; ask questions and
think carefully before agreeing to
surgery (rule 33), 42–45; ask
surgeon if they will use general or
local anesthetic (rule 47), 66–67;
ask surgeon to verify
anesthesiologist is board-certified
(rule 40), 54, 61; attempt to have
surgery in full-service hospital (rule
41), 54–55; avoid elective surgery
when residents and interns change
(rule 39), 53, 61; avoid travel far
away for a surgery from "best"
expert (rule 35), 46–49; be careful
about scheduling surgery "to avoid
losing time from work" if violates
other rules (rule 49), 68; consider
surgeon skilled in particular
surgery, even though they have
reputation for poor aftercare (rule
43), 58; do not have surgery on
holiday or weekend (rule 48),
67–68; don't panic if you must
violate some of rules 36-43 (rule
45), 63–65; let surgeon decide on
number of surgeries to be
performed (rule 50), 69–70; let
surgeon select method and
instruments of surgery (rule 46),
65–66; schedule elective surgery
for Monday, Tuesday, or
Wednesday morning (rule 38),
52–53; schedule surgery when

surgeon will be available seven days
postoperatively (rule 37), 51; select
surgeon carefully (rule 44), 59–63;
steps to assure best possible results
(rule 34), 45–46; verify with
surgeon that they will personally
perform the surgery (rule 36),
49–50

Safe Patients, Smart Hospitals, xxi
Sanders, Bernie, Senator, xxi, xxii
"schedule first" tips, 16–17
second opinions, xxiii, 13, 43, 44, 49,
108; during hospitalization, 98–99;
independent, 10–11, 43
skilled nursing facility (SNF), 47, 85
smartphones. *See* cell phones
SNF. *See* skilled nursing facility
Social Security, 131
specialists, 1, 21, 26, 155;
communication between, 37–39;
infectious disease, 52
spinal column, 150
spiral pad, 76, 99–100
state medical board, websites for, 5
statements, after injury, 144–146
stent, 78, 93
steroids, 119
supplements, 35–36
surgeon: acquaintance referrals for,
60; anesthetic choices of, 66–67;
avoiding travel for, 46–49; choice
of, 45, 57, 91–92; competent, 45,
47, 55, 59; computer search of, 60;
confirmation to perform surgery,
91–92; demeanor of, 62; dentures,
implants, or stents notification for,
93; experience of, 59, 61; follow-up
care from, 58; hospital choice of,
55; independent investigation of,
60; instrument choices of, 65–66;
insurance acceptance of, 60;
interview of, 61; methods of, 65–66;
number of procedures decided by,
69–70; postoperative availability of,

ABOUT THE AUTHORS

Robert M Fox, JD, received his BS in economics from the Wharton School of Finance of the University of Pennsylvania. He earned his law degree from Southwestern University and is engaged in the private practice of law in Sherman Oaks, California. He has a broad background in personal injury and medical malpractice, and his present legal affiliation is of counsel with Fox & Fox Law Corporation in Sherman Oaks (with James E. Fox). He is past president of the Los Angeles Trial Lawyers Association and the author of *The Medicolegal Report: Theory and Practice* as well as many medical-legal articles.

Chris Landon, MD, received his BS in psychobiology from the University of California and his medical degree from the University of Southern California. He was a pediatric intern and resident at Stanford University Hospital and received additional training at Stanford's Children's Hospital. He is board certified in both pediatrics and pediatric pulmonology and is director of pediatrics at Ventura County Medical Center. He is also clinical assistant professor of family medicine at UCLA and pediatrics at USC. He has contributed to articles in the *Journal of the American Medical Association*, the *Journal of the American Board of Family Practice*, and other professional publications and is the director of the Pediatric Diagnostic Center in Ventura, California.